Quality Assurance of Aseptic Preparation Services

Third edition

Edited by

Alison M Beaney

MSc, MRPharmS

Regional Quality Assurance Specialist
Pharmacy Department
Freeman Hospital
Newcastle upon Tyne, UK

on behalf of

The NHS QC Committee

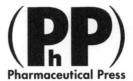

Pharmaceutical Press

Published by the Pharmaceutical Press
1 Lambeth High Street, London SE1 7JN, UK

© Pharmaceutical Press 2001

First edition published 1993 by the Quality Control Sub-Committee of the Regional
Pharmaceutical Officers Committee
Second edition published 1995 by the NHS QC Committee
Third edition published 2001 by the Pharmaceutical Press

Text design by Barker/Hilsdon, Lyme Regis, Dorset
Typeset by Mackreth Media Services, Hemel Hempstead, Hertfordshire
Printed in Great Britain by TJ International, Padstow, Cornwall

ISBN 0 85369 487 7

A catalogue record for this book is available from the British Library

Membership of the Quality Assurance of Aseptic Preparation Services Working Group

Alison Beaney, MSc, MRPharmS (Chairman)
Regional Quality Assurance Specialist
Northern & Yorkshire Region
Freeman Hospital, Newcastle upon Tyne, UK

Ian Beaumont, MRPharmS
Director of Quality Control
North-West Region
Stepping Hill Hospital, Stockport, UK

Paul Gurnell, MRPharmS
Principal Pharmacist
Aseptic Dispensing
Northern General Hospital, Sheffield, UK

Paul Maltby, MRPharmS
Principal Radiopharmacist
Royal Liverpool & Broadgreen University Hospitals, Liverpool, UK

Trevor Munton, PhD, MRPharmS
Regional Quality Assurance Officer
North Bristol NHS Trust
South & West Regional Health Authority, Bristol, UK

Richard Needle, PhD, MRPharmS
Chief Pharmacist
Colchester General Hospital, Colchester, UK

The Aseptic Services Working Group, comprising representatives from
the NHS Pharmaceutical Quality Control Committee and the NHS

Pharmaceutical Production Committee, was set up in 1994 under the Chairmanship of Dr M G Lee. The group produced the second edition of *The Quality Assurance of Aseptic Preparation Services* in 1995.

In 1998, a slightly differently constituted group reflecting the interest of smaller units and radiopharmacies was set up. Its aim was to produce standards for products for short-term use (up to 24 hours from preparation). These standards were published as a supplement to *The Quality Assurance of Aseptic Preparation Services*, 2nd edn, in 1999.

The members of both groups remaining in pharmaceutical services within the NHS were brought together in 1999 to produce this single consolidated standards book.

Contents

About the editor

Alison M Beaney (formerly Snowball) obtained a first class honours degree in Pharmacy at Sunderland School of Pharmacy in 1976, having been awarded the Hope Winch Scholarship in 1975. She completed her preregistration training at Newcastle General Hospital and registered in 1977.

After further study at Strathclyde University, she obtained an MSc in Pharmaceutical Analysis and began a career in hospital quality control at the Southern General Hospital in Glasgow.

She later returned to north-east England to take up the post of Quality Control Pharmacist at Freeman Hospital, and in 1991 was promoted to Regional Quality Assurance Specialist.

Alison has served as both secretary and chairman of the NHS Pharmaceutical Quality Control Committee and is also a member of numerous working groups of the committee. She took over chairmanship of the Aseptic Services Working Group in 1998, having been part of the group since 1993.

In addition, Alison is actively involved in the management and teaching of the Pharmaceutical Technology and Quality Assurance postgraduate course at Leeds University.

Preface

The Breckenridge Report, in 1976, recommended that preparation of intravenous injections should be carried out in pharmacy departments rather than on wards. Following this report, the NHS Pharmaceutical Quality Control Committee recognised the need for standards for aseptic preparation.

The first edition of *The Quality Assurance of Aseptic Preparation Services* was published in 1993. It was updated and expanded in 1995 to take account of recent publications including *Aseptic Dispensing for NHS Patients* (the Farwell report) and *Isolators for Pharmaceutical Applications*.

Aseptic preparation may be exempt from licensing provided certain criteria are met. One of these criteria is that all activities should be in accordance with defined NHS guidelines. The second edition of this booklet was recognised by the MCA and the Department of Health as the standard to which unlicensed aseptic units should be audited.

In 1996, ministers asked the MCA to audit a sample of unlicensed aseptic units in UK hospitals. The MCA reported that 60% of the units inspected had significant failings. This resulted in the issue of two Executive Letters on the subject of unlicensed aseptic preparation. The second of these Executive Letters, issued in August 1997, instigated a programme of external audit of NHS unlicensed aseptic preparation to be undertaken by regional quality assurance specialists, in collaboration with regional offices.

Audits identified the need for standards for products for short-term use (up to 24 hours from preparation). As a result, standards for this activity were published as a supplement to the second edition of *The Quality Assurance of Aseptic Preparation Services* in July 1999. Publication of this third edition allows both standards to be presented in a single consolidated document which also incorporates a number of additions and amendments to reflect current practice.

The Editor would like to thank all members of the Aseptic Services Working Group, both past and present, for their hard work and conscientiousness in preparing these standards. She would also like to acknowledge the helpful comments received from the NHS Pharmaceutical Quality Control Committee, the UK Radiopharmacy Group, and the NHS Production Committee.

Alison M Beaney
March 2001

Acknowledgements

We would like to acknowledge the contributions of Rob Duncombe and the National CIVAS Group for Appendix 2, section A2.2 (operator validation test) and Rob Duncombe and Stephen Langford for assistance with Appendix 2, section A2.7 (computer validation). Thanks also to Mike Lillywhite for contributing Appendix 5 and to Lynn Harrison for typing the manuscript.

1

Introduction

As far back as 1976, the Breckenridge report[1] recommended that drug additions to intravenous infusions should be made in pharmacy departments and not on wards, advice which is retained in the current *British National Formulary* (BNF). The first edition of *The Quality Assurance of Aseptic Preparation Services*, published in January 1993, gave advice and guidance on the quality assurance procedures that are necessary to ensure the quality of products prepared aseptically in hospitals.[2] It was produced as a result of the requirement, in the Medicines Control Agency (MCA) document *Guidance to the NHS on the Licensing Requirements of the Medicines Act 1968*,[3] for defined National Health Service (NHS) guidelines. An updated and expanded edition was published in 1995.[4] This current edition has been further updated to reflect recent changes in NHS practice.

The MCA guidance[3] defines dispensing as 'the activity of supplying the product in its appropriate form to the patient pursuant to a doctor's prescription.' Activities that take place prior to the act of supply are considered to be preparation, assembly or manufacture.

Preparation is exempt from the licensing requirements of the Medicines Act[5] and includes preparation for individual patients and preparation of stock from which to dispense to individual patients in accordance with a prescription. Nevertheless the MCA guidance placed certain restrictions on preparation for stock and these have been extended by the Farwell report[6] to cover preparation for dispensing directly to individual patients. The conditions specified by the MCA are as follows:

Aseptic preparation is exempt from the licensing requirements of the Medicines Act provided all the following conditions are met:

1. The preparation is done by or under the supervision of a pharmacist, who takes full responsibility for the quality of the product.
2. The preparation uses closed systems.
3. Licensed sterile medicinal products are used as ingredients or the ingredients are manufactured sterile in licensed facilities.

4. Products will be allocated a shelf-life of no more than 1 week. The shelf-life should be supported by stability data.
5. All activities should be in accordance with defined NHS guidelines.

Preparation activities meeting the above criteria will require an acceptable level of quality assurance together with regular external audit by quality assurance staff.

These guidelines are applicable to all products prepared aseptically for administration to patients. Total parenteral nutrition (TPN) solutions, cytotoxic injections, radiopharmaceuticals and additives for parenteral administration are the most common examples of such products but other dosage forms, e.g. irrigations, complying with the above criteria are also affected.

It is not the intention of this book to cause pharmacy-based activities to cease, with reversion of this work to lower standard conditions at ward level. However, since patient safety is of paramount importance, units should continually review their facilities and quality assurance procedures to ensure that standards of quality are being maintained. Should circumstances arise where this is no longer the case, a risk assessment should be carried out (see Chapter 3).

In 1996, the government asked the MCA to audit a 10% sample of the unlicensed aseptic units in UK hospitals. The MCA reported that 60% of the units inspected had significant failings. As a result *Executive Letter (96) 95*[7] was issued in December 1996. This required all units undertaking non-licensed aseptic preparation to carry out an internal audit of their activities and standards. The outcomes of this audit were summarised in August 1997 in *Executive Letter (97) 52*,[8] which additionally required a programme of external audit of NHS unlicensed aseptic preparation to be undertaken by regional quality assurance specialists in collaboration with the performance management arm of regional offices. At the time of going to press, aseptic preparation remains exempt from licensing if the five conditions stated earlier apply. However, these conditions are currently under review by the MCA. Trusts have a legal obligation to ensure that any unlicensed aseptic preparation complies with published standards and are liable to prosecution under the Medicines Act if medicinal products they prepare are not of the nature or quality intended.

The need for standards for products for short-term use (up to 24 hours from preparation) was identified by the results of the audits carried out under *Executive Letter (96) 95*.[7] These were published as a supplement to the second edition of *The Quality Assurance of Aseptic Preparation Services* in July 1999.[9] There has now been time for these standards to be applied in practice and re-evaluated. Publication of this third edition allows both standards to be put into context by their incorporation into this single consolidated book.

Since the last edition of this book was published, a new version of *Rules and Guidance for Pharmaceutical Manufacturers and Distributors*[10] has been published which gives more detailed standards, for example for the environment. This new edition incorporates these standards and is more prescriptive in many ways than its forerunner. Within this edition there is also increased emphasis on training and competency assessment, to reflect commitment to continuous professional development.

In 1997, the Department of Health published *The New NHS: Modern, Dependable*,[11] which introduced the concept of clinical governance and emphasised the importance of setting and promoting quality standards. A second government policy document, *A First Class Service – Quality in the New NHS*,[12] referred to the setting of clear national standards and the need for consistent monitoring arrangements. Although these documents were aimed at the clinical situation, the principles are equally relevant in the sphere of pharmacy technical services. Clinical governance must, however, balance the need for accountability and the highest standards of practice from all staff, with the need to preserve and enhance the ability of the NHS to meet the needs and expectations of patients as fully as possible.

Standards underpin the audit process, and the review of this standards document effectively closes the audit loop initiated in 1995 by publication of the second edition and implemented by *Executive Letter (96) 95*.[7] The series of controls assurance documents[13] introduced in 2000 indicates the high level of commitment to the audit culture within the NHS. This new edition is an essential part of medicines management and should ensure that non-licensed aseptic preparation lies within the NHS continuing quality improvement framework.

2

Definitions

2.1 Authorised pharmacist

This is the person designated in writing by the responsible pharmacist to supervise the aseptic process and release the product for use.

2.2 Chief pharmacist

This is the pharmacist responsible for the pharmacy services within a corporate body. In the context of this book, for aseptic facilities not under the direct management control of the chief pharmacist, this responsibility lies with the most senior pharmacist.

2.3 Clean room

A clean room is a room in which the number and concentration of viable and non-viable airborne particles is controlled. The room is constructed and used in a manner that minimises the introduction, generation and retention of particles inside the room, and other relevant parameters, e.g. temperature and humidity, are controlled as necessary.

2.4 Closed procedure

A closed procedure is a procedure whereby a sterile pharmaceutical is prepared by transferring sterile ingredients or solutions to a pre-sterilised sealed container, either directly or using a sterile transfer device, without exposing the solution to the external environment.

The use of a solution from a sealed ampoule can be regarded as a closed procedure when a single withdrawal is made from the ampoule, immediately after opening, using a sterile syringe and needle or equivalent device.

The above assumes that, for aseptic preparation and dispensing activities, all closed procedures are performed within a European Union Good Manufacturing Practice (EU GMP) grade A environment.

2.5 Controlled workspace

A controlled workspace is an enclosed workspace constructed and operated in such a manner and equipped with appropriate air-handling and filtration systems to reduce to a predefined level the introduction, generation and retention of contaminants.

2.6 Critical zone

The critical zone is that part of the controlled workspace where containers are opened and the product is exposed. Particulate and microbiological contamination should be reduced to levels appropriate to the intended use.

2.7 External audit

An external audit is undertaken by staff who are not managerially accountable within the corporate structure in which the aseptic preparation unit is situated, and are independent of any service provision to the unit.

2.8 High Efficiency Particulate Air (HEPA) filters

These are filters with classification no less than H13 when tested according to EN 1822.[14]

2.9 Immediate use

Products prepared under uncontrolled conditions are for immediate use and administration should commence as soon as practicable after preparation has been completed. The time of preparation is considered to be the time when the sterile seal of the primary packaging is breached.

2.10 Internal audit

An internal audit is undertaken by staff who are a part of the management organisational structure of the department.

2.11 Pharmaceutical isolator

A pharmaceutical isolator is a containment device that utilises barrier technology for the enclosure of a controlled workspace.

2.12 Pharmaceutical isolator transfer device

This is a device, which can be fixed or removable, that allows material to be transferred into and out of the pharmaceutical isolator.

2.13 Primary packaging

This is the packaging that immediately encloses a single unit. In the case of a sterile component the primary packaging will maintain the sterility of the individual unit.

2.14 Quality assurance officer

The quality assurance officer's responsibilities include:

- providing advice on procedures and techniques (in conjunction with the responsible pharmacist where appropriate)
- providing advice on documentation
- making regular visits to the unit for general quality assurance purposes
- ensuring the provision of an agreed environmental monitoring (including commissioning) and microbiological testing service, monitoring the results obtained and discussing any problems with the responsible pharmacist and the regional quality assurance pharmacist if appropriate.

In addition, the quality assurance officer should be able to provide or arrange an analytical testing service and assist in self-inspection if required.

2.15 Quality exception report

A quality exception report is a report of any deviation from standard procedures and documentation that occurs during the preparation process and consequent remedial action.

2.16 Responsible pharmacist

This is the pharmacist responsible for all aspects of the services within an aseptic preparation unit. The duties of the responsible pharmacist include the approval of all systems of work and documentation used in the unit. This person is also an authorised pharmacist.

2.17 Secondary packaging

This is the packaging that encloses multiples of individual units. The secondary packaging may be removed without affecting the characteristics of the product, e.g. loss of sterility.

In the context in which the term is used in this book any packaging that encloses, for example, a single ampoule or vial is considered to be secondary packaging.

2.18 Short-term use

Products for short-term use should commence administration within 24 hours of preparation on condition that stability data is satisfactory. They will have been prepared under controlled conditions complying with the guidance in Appendix 4.

2.19 Standard operating procedures

Standard operating procedures are detailed written documents formally approved by the responsible pharmacist. They describe the operations to be carried out, the precautions to be taken and the measures to be applied that are directly or indirectly related to the preparation and supply of the product. They give directions for performing certain operations, e.g. cleaning, changing, environmental monitoring and equipment operation, to ensure that they are performed to a consistent standard.

2.20   Supervision

The pharmacist responsible for supervision should be in the department and in a position to intervene at any part of the aseptic preparation process. He/she should be aware of what is going on and be able to ensure that the process is carried out in the prescribed manner.

In practice this requires the pharmacist to:

- be fully conversant with all approved systems of work and documentation associated with the aseptic preparation process, from prescription verification to issue of the product
- verify all prescriptions before preparation commences
- perform final checking (including checking against the prescription) of all products prepared, and release them for issue.

2.21   Support room

The support room is a dedicated room that is used for activities that are ancillary to the aseptic preparation process. Such activities may include component assembly, generation of documentation, labelling, checking and packaging.

3

Risk management

3.1 Introduction

This section gives guidance on the risks associated with the aseptic preparation of medicines, and on the assessment and management of these risks.

3.2 The risks

3.2.1 Medication errors

Medication errors can result in patient mortality and morbidity, and need to be prevented. A series of articles published each month since 1993 in *Pharmacy in Practice* has described serious medication errors and methods of avoiding these incidents. A summary of parenteral medication errors was published in 1997.[15] Frequently described medication errors result from the following:

- incorrect dosage calculations by medical and nursing staff
- incorrect drug product, dose and diluent selection
- incorrect preparation method
- absence of product labelling and documentation of parenterals prepared at ward or theatre level
- incorrect route and method of administration
- incorrect operation of parenteral infusion pumps.

Many of the above errors have been repeated in hospitals throughout the UK on several occasions. Reports from hospitals indicate that the clinical workload has significantly increased in recent years and at the same time the number of suitably trained doctors and nurses on the wards who are able to carry out the preparation of parenteral medicines has decreased. The increased workload has also changed the ward environment, making it very difficult for ward staff to prepare parenteral medicines in an appropriate environment without constant interruption.

3.2.2   Microbiological contamination

For aseptically prepared products there are five major sources of contamination:

- airborne contamination
- contamination by touch
- surface contamination of components
- contamination during storage
- contamination during administration.

The risk of contamination is dependent on a number of key factors, which are listed below:

The aseptic technique of the operator   As only closed procedures are used, the most likely route of contamination of the product (other than due to any inherent contamination of components) is faulty aseptic technique. The training of operators is a critical aspect of aseptic processing and must be supported by regular validation of technique.

Aseptic workspace   The more viable organisms there are in the immediate environment of the process at the point the container is breached, the greater the risk that some will enter the sterile product. Environmental standards, and the monitoring of those standards, are therefore a fundamental part of every quality assurance system.

Open or closed procedures   Closed transfer procedures between two sealed containers using an integrated transfer device have a far lower risk of contamination when compared to an open procedure in which the sterile container is open to the atmosphere, albeit for a few seconds. For open procedures, the standard of environment at the point of fill is particularly critical.

3.2.2.1   Risk of infection

Data have been published relating propofol usage to the occurrence of post-operative infection. In these reports the risk factors leading to post-operative infection were identified as poor aseptic technique, prolonged infusion times, preparation of multiple syringes and prolonged storage of opened ampoules.[16-18] As a result of these and similar findings, it is now recommended that the dose be prepared just prior to administration and that the infusion be completed within 6 hours of the ampoule or vial being opened. However, in some circumstances 6 hours may be too long, especially for preparations such as propofol that support microbial growth. A more recent study found that times exceeding 95 minutes between drawing up and administration of propofol were associated with systemic infections.[19]

3.2.2.2   Contamination rates in uncontrolled environments

The risk of contamination is far higher when injections are prepared in uncontrolled environments. Furthermore, the risk of contamination increases as the number of additions made to the infusion increases. Contamination rates of up to 5% have been reported in infusion fluids to which no additives have been made.[20–23] This rate can increase to 50% following addition to the solutions.[22–24] In all of these studies, fluids were tested retrospectively after administration. As an example of the long-term consequences of these contamination rates, it has been reported that 42% of patients in an intensive care unit were found to have an extrinsically contaminated intravenous administration system at least once during a three-month period.[25]

All the above data refer to products prepared in unclassified environments in ward areas or intensive care units. As such, they are indicators of contamination rates for products prepared in these uncontrolled areas. It is not possible, however, to relate the data to infection frequency.

3.3   Management of the risks

3.3.1   Conducting risk assessments and option appraisals

In order to minimise the risks of microbiological contamination and medication errors associated with the preparation of parenteral medication at ward level, it is always preferable to perform the aseptic preparation of medicines within suitable facilities under the control of a pharmacist.[8] However, this is not always possible. Risk management, involving risk assessments and option appraisals, should be performed on all aseptic preparation activities carried out within hospital trusts.

One of the methodologies for risk assessment that is gaining favour in the pharmaceutical industry is the use of hazard analysis and critical control points (HACCP).[26] This approach examines each step in the process and identifies potential hazards – creating a flow chart is the first stage. Having identified the risks, it is then possible to assess whether these are adequately controlled at that point or at a later stage in the process.

Another essential requirement is to have systems in place which ensure that lessons are learned from mistakes. Error reporting, early warning systems (near misses), along with a no-blame culture, are the principles of clinical governance.[27]

The following steps may be used as a framework for risk assessment:

1. Gather information
   (i) Products, presentations and numbers.
   (ii) Staff grades undertaking aseptic manipulations.
   (iii) Types of manipulations undertaken.
   (iv) Areas where activities occur.
   (v) Times when aseptic preparation occurs.
   (vi) Training programmes in place.

2. Assess against standards
   (i) Training and competencies of individuals involved.
   (ii) Suitability of environment in which these activities occur.
   (iii) Actual practice for preparation of products.

3. Identify action
   (i) Identify activities that should be carried out under pharmacy control.
   (ii) Prioritise these activities and prepare action plan.
   (iii) Identify which products should be prepared in-house and which should be out-sourced.
   (iv) Identify activities that should be carried out in clinical areas.
   (v) Identify any action required to bring these activities up to the required standard.

Factors influencing where products need to be prepared, and by whom, include:

- the complexity of the preparation process and the risk of preparation error (e.g. incorrect calculation or dilution)
- the potential for the contamination of the product
- the potential for microbial growth in the finished product
- the health and safety risks to persons preparing and handling the product

- the potential for incompatibility
- the chemical stability of the product
- the duration of the infusion
- other pharmaceutical considerations (e.g. the packaging system)
- regulatory requirements
- the need for urgency in the supply of the product
- clinical issues, e.g. the clinical condition of patients receiving the product.

Where a product requires reconstitution, consideration must be given to the final form in which the product will be delivered.

For individual product types, examples of their more specific risk factors are:

- *cytotoxics/radiopharmaceuticals:* high level of hazard to the operator preparing the product and high risk of preparation errors
- *parenteral nutrition (PN) solutions:* may be very complex; high risk of microbial contamination and high risk of preparation error
- *epidurals/cardioplegia solutions:* high risk associated with microbial contamination
- *infusors/ambulatory devices (e.g. infusor and patient-controlled analgesia):* risk of microbial growth; some products may be administered over significant periods of time at temperatures at or near body temperature during administration; technical complexity
- *syringes, minibags and infusions:* risk of preparation errors and microbial contamination; some solutions may promote bacterial and/or fungal growth; some solutions may be administered over significant lengths of time
- *irrigations (excluding ophthalmic):* immediacy of use, or otherwise
- *eye preparations (unpreserved or preserved):* risk of microbial growth; complexity; risk of preparation error
- *others (e.g. biologicals, factor VIII):* must be assessed on an individual product basis.

Note: The lowest risk of microbial contamination is with products that are administered directly from the licensed container, or products not requiring reconstitution, that are withdrawn immediately prior to administration from a unit dose container (e.g. vial or ampoule) or a licensed multidose vial containing antimicrobial preservative.

3.3.2 Controlling where and by whom preparation takes place

The options for the location of aseptic preparation are:

1. an uncontrolled area in a ward, clinic or theatre
2. a dedicated room or facility with no pharmaceutical isolator
3. a dedicated room or facility containing a pharmaceutical isolator (satellite unit)
4. a dedicated facility containing a laminar flow cabinet in a clean room complying with the standards of Chapter 6
5. a centralised pharmacy aseptic unit.

1. This carries the highest risks of both microbial contamination and preparation errors. Recent work has shown high levels of airborne micro-organisms in this type of area, resulting in an increased probability of ingress of viable micro-organisms during the preparation process.[28] The absence of controlled standard operating procedures, documentation, appropriate staff training, monitoring and checking, and the distractions of the busy ward environment all contribute significantly to the risk of preparation errors.

2. The availability of a dedicated area in the ward or clinical area for the preparation of injections may go some way towards reducing the risks of preparation errors, but in order to minimise these risks it would be necessary to establish procedural and documentation controls, under the supervision of a pharmacist, which fully comply with the good practice requirements of this book. The high risk of microbial contamination during preparation would remain, resulting in a requirement for any product prepared in this type of environment to be used immediately.

3. The use of this type of facility provides a significantly lower risk of microbial contamination than the previous areas. Again, controls complying with good practice requirements and under the supervision of a pharmacist on staff training and monitoring, standard operating procedures and documentation are required to minimise preparation errors.

Such a facility would be expected to comply with the standards in Appendix 4.

4. The use of this type of facility provides a reduced level of risk that is similar to 3 above. Compliance with the NHS quality assurance guidelines may be more difficult in a satellite setting, and this type of facility is best accommodated in a centralised unit.

5.   These units carry the least risk of contamination or preparation errors and are recommended for all aseptic preparation operations.

Risks of microbial contamination and medication errors can be eliminated, or significantly reduced, by involving the hospital pharmacy service more closely in the preparation and supply of sterile solutions in a ready-to-administer form, and supplementing this supply service with input from clinical pharmacists. The preparation of these solutions in pharmacy-controlled centralised or satellite units places the responsibility with health professionals, who have the necessary education and training to enable them to provide a safe and appropriate therapy to hospital patients.

Each circumstance will be different and requires risk assessment using professional judgements. These assessments should take account of:

- the increased rate of microbiological contamination for additives prepared in uncontrolled environments
- the higher levels of microbial contaminants in uncontrolled environments
- the increased risk of systemic infection associated with products prepared in uncontrolled environments
- the increased risk of medication errors when preparing injections without pharmacy supervision.

Evaluation of the options currently available for the aseptic preparation of unpreserved injections shows that the preferred option is for them to be prepared in a pharmacy-controlled, validated aseptic unit. When prepared outside pharmacy control they should be administered immediately, as recommended in the Committee for Proprietary Medicinal Products (CPMP) guidelines.[29]

3.3.3   Limiting the shelf-lives of products prepared

Limiting the shelf-life of medicinal products is intended to ensure that product quality is maintained in the period between preparation and complete administration. For aseptically prepared products, the generally accepted criteria are that at the time of administration the product is sterile and contains not less than 90% of the stated content of the active ingredient. The expiry period is therefore determined by the physico-chemical stability of the product and by the risk of microbiological contamination during preparation and administration.

3.3.3.1 Physico-chemical stability

The factors affecting physico-chemical stability are well known and well documented. They include storage temperature, pH, drug concentrations and the infusion fluid used as the vehicle. Chapter 5 contains a more complete discussion of these factors. For many products, literature evidence is now available on their physico-chemical stability. Furthermore, it is possible to carry out laboratory investigations to justify or validate expiry dates. Since physico-chemical stability is related to the chemical properties of the individual compounds and is not affected by the preparation process, it is possible to predict or determine the time for 10% degradation to occur (or the time for unacceptable levels of breakdown products to occur) and relate this to the storage temperature of the prepared product.

3.3.3.2 Contamination and infection

Assigning a shelf-life solely on the basis of the risk of microbiological contamination is not possible: either a product is sterile or it is not. Furthermore, it does not necessarily follow that infection will result from the administration of a contaminated injection, since the normal human immune system can usually inactivate small numbers of viable organisms and so prevent serious infection. The following factors also need to be considered.

Antibacterial properties of the injection Antibiotic infusions and preserved injections have a known bacterial activity against a specific spectrum of micro-organisms. There is evidence that some radiopharmaceutical preparations have anti-bacterial properties.[30, 31] However, although similar claims are made for cytotoxic agents, research shows that cytotoxic preparations may support or enhance the survival of micro-organisms.[32] On the basis of these data it cannot be assumed that any injection solution is self-sterilising.

Storage temperature The optimum incubation temperatures for the majority of micro-organisms are in the range 25–35°C. At refrigerator temperatures (2–8°C), growth will usually be retarded or stopped.[33] However, when contaminated products are moved from the refrigerator to room or body temperature, organisms will begin to grow after a recovery lag period of a few hours.

Growth characteristics of micro-organisms   There is a lag time before any contaminating organisms begin to grow and proliferate. This lag time is longer for damaged cells in a nutrient-deficient medium. Biological variability is such, however, that it is not possible to make accurate predictions for specific infusion fluids.

3.3.3.3 Current legislation and guidelines relating to product shelf-life

The Medicines Act 1968[5]   There are no shelf-lives quoted in The Medicines Act 1968. The Act lays down controls of licensed medicinal products. Expiry periods are evaluated as part of the licence application documentation.

Subject to satisfactory chemical stability data, injections that are supplied as sterile dry powders are recommended to be used within 24 hours of reconstitution. This recommendation is included in the product data sheet and is a condition of the product licence.

MCA guidance on the application of the Medicines Act 1968 to NHS hospitals[3]   The MCA guidelines state that aseptically prepared products should have a maximum 7-day shelf-life. When the document was issued, the limit of 7 days was arbitrarily set as a shelf-life that would allow hospital aseptic units to operate economically and develop centralised services, but it was recognised that this would restrict the numbers of products prepared.

Expiry periods given to products must be evaluated in accordance with local conditions and as a general principle the shortest expiry consistent with the intended usage pattern of the product should be used. See Chapter 5 for guidance on in-use storage times.

Committee for Proprietary Medicinal Products   The CPMP is responsible for the provision of advice to the pharmaceutical industry on product licence applications and the registration of medicinal products. It is a committee of the Directorate General III of the European Commission. In a guidance note on the maximum shelf-life for sterile products after first opening or following reconstitution,[30] it makes the following recommendation:

'From a microbiological point of view, the product should be used immediately. If not used immediately, in-use storage times and conditions prior to use are the responsibility of the user and would normally be not longer than 24 hours at 2–8°C, unless reconstitution/dilution/opening has taken place in controlled and validated aseptic conditions.'

British National Formulary[34]   The BNF currently recommends that because of the risk of microbial contamination to intravenous additives, a maximum shelf-life of 12 hours should be imposed for additions made other than in a pharmacy-run aseptic preparation unit.

Shelf-lives of 24 hours and less are intended to reduce the risk to the patient in the event of an injection becoming contaminated during preparation. However, there is no scientific evidence to support or justify any shelf-life on the basis of the risk of patient infection. From the foregoing discussion the following key points must always be taken into consideration when determining the site of preparation, and storage time and temperature prior to use:

- there is an increased risk of contamination for products prepared in uncontrolled environments
- products prepared in uncontrolled environments should not be stored at room temperature for a period of time that might allow proliferation of micro-organisms.

4

Management

4.1 Principle

Aseptic preparation departments must ensure that the products they supply are fit for their intended use and do not place patients at risk. Achieving this objective is the responsibility of pharmacy managers and requires the commitment, understanding and participation of all staff who are involved in the ordering, preparation, storage and supply of aseptic products. There must be a comprehensive and correctly implemented system of quality assurance incorporating the principles of GMP[10] and standards for dispensing procedures.[35] The system should be fully documented and its effectiveness monitored.

4.2 Recommendations

(a) All departments undertaking aseptic preparation activities should have a documented organisational structure that indicates clearly the responsibilities and accountability of each member of staff.

(b) The quality assurance system must be fully documented and units should continually review their quality assurance procedures to ensure that standards of quality are maintained. Should circumstances arise where this is no longer the case, the work must cease and contingency plans should be implemented.

(c) There should be a detailed contingency plan to cover any unforeseen shutdown of the unit or any temporary unavailability of the service. The use of alternative aseptic facilities should be identified and the risks assessed. Service level reductions, or a review of shelf-life and storage conditions, may be necessary to reduce the risk.

(d) It is the responsibility of the chief pharmacist to ensure that internal audits of aseptic preparation are carried out on a regular basis, that quality assurance systems are regularly reviewed and that off-site testing is regularly audited. Any faults or deficiencies, however identified, must be promptly rectified.

(e) The chief pharmacist should ensure that the department has a current capacity plan (see Appendix 5). Workload figures should be regularly reviewed against this plan and action taken where appropriate.

(f) It is the responsibility of regional quality assurance specialists to ensure that external audits are carried out in accordance with current NHS requirements.[8]

(g) Aseptic units must be under the management of a responsible pharmacist who must ensure that a system of quality assurance is implemented that incorporates the principles set down in this book. Routine monitoring of the adherence to procedures in the form of self-inspection should be undertaken.

(h) All aseptic preparation must be carried out by or under the supervision of a pharmacist authorised by the responsible pharmacist. (The responsible pharmacist is also an authorised pharmacist by definition.) Pharmacists supervising any aseptic preparation carried out outside normal working hours must be authorised pharmacists.

(i) The responsibility for the release of an aseptically prepared product must be taken by an authorised pharmacist in accordance with the criteria set down in Chapter 13. This may not necessarily be the same authorised pharmacist who supervised the preparation of the product.

(j) The responsible pharmacist should authorise the standard operating procedures. Any deviation from these procedures must be approved by the responsible or authorised pharmacist supervising at the time and should be fully documented.

(k) All staff who are involved in the preparation and supply of aseptically prepared products should clearly understand their level of responsibility and accountability, and should complete an appropriate programme of training.

(l) The decision on which products are to be regularly prepared should be made by the responsible pharmacist, who will carry out a risk assessment (see Chapter 3).

(m)   The responsible pharmacist should authorise documented procedures for regularly prepared products and these procedures should be readily available. These procedures should be based on evaluated data but if no data are available the decision to prepare the product should be made in the context of the clinical needs of the patient and the potential risks.

(n)   When an authorised pharmacist decides, using the criteria in Chapter 3, to prepare a product for which there are no documented procedures, he/she takes full responsibility for the quality of that product and the procedures used for preparation must be fully documented.

5

Formulation, stability and shelf-life

5.1   Introduction

Expiry periods given to products must be evaluated in accordance with the local conditions. Data obtained from the literature or from the manufacturer should be carefully assessed to ensure their appropriateness. The overall aim must be to minimise the time between preparation of the product and its administration so that the opportunity for any live micro-organisms in the product to multiply is restricted. As a general principle, the shortest expiry period consistent with the intended usage pattern of the product should be used. Under no circumstances should an expiry period of 7 days be exceeded for products prepared in unlicensed units (see Chapter 3). Use of the shortest possible shelf-life does not obviate the need to comply fully with the standards described in this book.

The range of formulations encountered during aseptic preparation is immense and ranges from fairly simple two-component systems to complex mixtures with in excess of 50 components, e.g. PN regimen.

Stability should be assessed to ensure the quality of the product is suitable for the patient at the time of administration. However, no ͏ ͏ rule exists to assess stability.

gradation

hanisms of chemical degradation are hydrolysis, oxida-ɔlysis. Other degradation pathways, e.g. polymerisation tion, can also occur.

rs affecting stability

he ingredients, a number of other factors can affect stability.

5.3.1   Concentration of active components

Concentration can either enhance or reduce stability, e.g. ampicillin degrades more quickly in high concentrations than in dilute solutions. Oxidation and photodegradation can be more significant at lower concentrations.

5.3.2   Ionic strength

An example of the effect of ionic strength is cisplatin in solution, which is stabilised by the presence of chloride ion and requires sodium chloride, for example, at a concentration of at least 0.3% w/v.

5.3.3   pH

The rates of hydrolysis of many drugs are pH dependent. For example, amphotericin in glucose 5% infusion requires a pH of greater than 4.2 to be stable.

5.3.4   Vehicle

Erythromycin injection can be diluted in sodium chloride 0.9% or glucose 5% but is more stable in sodium chloride than in glucose.

5.3.5   Catalysis

Some ingredients in formulations can act as catalysts for the breakdown of other ingredients, e.g. copper ions from trace metal additions in PN preparations catalyse the degradation of ascorbic acid.

5.3.6   Preparation process

Production methodology can be critical. The correct order of mixing of materials in PN compounding is essential to avoid high concentrations of electrolytes, which affect lipid particle size, and also to avoid high concentrations of metal ions mixing with phosphate, which could cause precipitation.

5.3.7   Photosensitivity

Some chemicals are sensitive to light. There can be significant photodegradation of drugs, e.g. carmustine, amphotericin and some vitamins.

5.3.8 Filters

Filters used in production processes can cause problems. Adsorption onto the filter medium will reduce the potency of some injections (e.g. epoprostenol onto standard cellulose ester membranes). Similarly, some apparent solutions are in fact colloids, e.g. amphotericin, for which a filter pore size of 1 μm or greater is required.

5.3.9 Containers

The nature of the container can contribute to stability problems by interacting with the product, by releasing chemicals (e.g. plasticiser from PVC bags) or by adsorption of ingredients from the solution onto the container. Much of the quoted work on carmustine is in glass containers for this reason. Paclitaxel (Taxol) also requires presentation in glass or polyolefin infusion containers. Container permeability should also be considered; gaseous diffusion into the container or drug loss due to absorption and permeation through the plastic can cause problems.

5.3.10 Storage

In general, low storage temperatures slow down chemical degradation, adsorption, etc. However, it should be remembered that low-temperature storage can result in physical instability, e.g. precipitation, such as in aciclovir infusions. However, the converse can also be true: phosphates are less soluble at room or body temperature, which has led to precipitation in PN solution.

5.3.11 Duration of storage

Prolonged storage can reveal the effects of a number of routes of degradation. Products become unsuitable for use where they are physically unsuitable, e.g. precipitation and discoloration, the active component degrades or breakdown products form to an unacceptable degree.

5.4 Sources of information

Many sources of information about stability exist, but it is the responsibility of the authorised pharmacist to ensure that the information used is scientifically valid and that it actually applies to the local circumstances, bearing in mind the points made above.

A number of texts are available through quality control pharmacists and medicines information, including the UK stability database, textbooks, product data sheets and published research papers. Product manufacturers are a prime source of information, particularly in respect of PN.

Suitable data should be sought and evaluated before products are prepared. If no data are available the decision to prepare should be made in the context of the clinical needs of the patient.

5.5 Injection preparation

Aseptic preparation facilities in many hospital pharmacies now enable the preparation of injections in controlled environments where the sterility of the product can be assured. Under these circumstances and where the starting material is a licensed product or has been prepared in a licensed unit and the sterile medication is prepared under conditions of GMP in suitably audited premises, then the expiry date allocated may give due consideration to both the chemical properties of the preparation and the microbiological integrity of the process and product, up to a maximum of 7 days (see Chapter 3).

5.6 Shelf-life

The shelf-life should reflect the intended use and administration of the product and should take account of, for example, prolonged storage at skin or body temperature.

Facilities

6.1 Facilities – general issues

(a)   The performance criteria of the facility should be established prior to building. Adherence to the design specification should be demonstrated by monitoring of the facility at commissioning and during use.[36, 37]

(b)   All aseptic operations should be performed in a workstation sited as recommended in sections 6.2 and 6.3, and with a controlled workspace environment conforming to EU Guide grade A.[10] This may be provided by:

- a laminar flow cabinet
- a pharmaceutical isolator.

For products for short-term use see Appendix 4.

(c)   Ideally, clean-air devices should run continuously. Should it be necessary to switch off the device, e.g. for cleaning or maintenance purposes, aseptic manipulation should not be carried out until a satisfactory environment has been achieved, as demonstrated by appropriate validation studies.

(d)   Pressure differentials across inlet HEPA filters in cabinets, isolators and clean rooms, and between rooms of different classification should be constantly indicated. There should be alarms to indicate malfunction. Pressure differentials should be recorded at defined intervals.

(e)   All rooms and equipment used for preparation activities should be cleaned regularly and frequently in accordance with an agreed written procedure. The procedure should require written confirmation that cleaning has been carried out.

(f) All equipment should be operated in accordance with written operating instructions. Major equipment, including air-handling systems, should be subject to a suitable planned preventative maintenance schedule.

(g) All aseptic preparation facilities should be commissioned by quality control and then monitored at regular intervals (see section 10.2). When monitoring indicates a loss of environmental control, the reasons for loss of control should be determined and remedial action taken. Recommissioning may be necessary.

6.2 Laminar flow cabinets

(a) Laminar flow cabinets must be situated in a clean room that is dedicated to aseptic preparation. The room environment must comply with EU Guide grade B.[10] The siting of the cabinet within the room is crucial to the cabinet's correct function.

(b) Airflow patterns in the clean room and in the cabinets should not create any dead spots or standing vortices. Determination of airflow patterns should be carried out on commissioning and after any significant modification to the room or cabinet.

(c) The construction of the clean room should comply with EU GMP requirements. These recommend that walls, floor and ceiling should be smooth and impervious to allow cleaning; bare wood and other unsealed surfaces must be avoided. To reduce dust accumulation and facilitate cleaning there should be a minimum of shelves and other projecting fittings. The junctions of walls, floor and ceiling should be coved. The room must not contain a sink.

(d) The clean room must be entered through a changing room. Changing rooms should be designed as airlocks and used to provide separation of the different stages of change and so minimise microbial and particulate contamination of protective clothing.

(e) The final stage of the changing room should not contain a sink. A social hand wash prior to entry to the room followed by a disinfectant hand rub at the point of gloving is recommended. Hand-washing facilities and the water supplied to them should be regularly monitored for compliance with appropriate limits (e.g. the EU limits for potable water are 100 cfu/mL at 25°C and 10 cfu/mL at 35°C).

(f)   Sterilised clean-room clothing should be worn by all staff entering the room. Alternative methods that guarantee the clothing is initially free from viable organisms may be used, e.g. a validated biocidal wash. Levels of particulate contamination should also be controlled.

(g)   All points of access to and egress from the room should be fitted with an interlocked or alarmed door system.

(h)   There should be a support room from which materials can be passed into and out of the clean room through a hatch(es). The doors of the hatch(es) should be interlocked.

(i)   A validated transfer process should be used to transfer materials into the clean room.

6.3   Pharmaceutical isolators

(a)   Isolators should be sited in a dedicated room used only for the isolator and its ancillary equipment and related activities. The interior surfaces of the room (walls, floor, ceiling) should be smooth and free from cracks and open joints. They should not shed particulate matter and should allow easy and effective cleaning and sanitation.

(b)   The background environment in which the isolator is sited should comply with the air quality category defined in *Isolators for Pharmaceutical Applications*[38] in accordance with the type of isolator and its transfer system. Currently EU GMP requirements[10] state that isolators for aseptic processing should be sited in a minimum grade D environment.

(c)   Siting and use of sinks should be carefully considered in view of their potential to cause microbiological contamination. Sinks or handwashing facilities should not be available inside isolator rooms, to prevent aerosol or liquid sprays impinging on the materials being processed. However, if after careful consideration these facilities are considered essential in adjacent areas, they must be regularly monitored and disinfected.

(d)   Access to the room should be restricted to authorised personnel. During use only those people who are actively involved in the process should be in the room.

(e)   The design of the isolator should follow the principles laid down in *Isolators for Pharmaceutical Applications*.[38]

(f)   All aseptic manipulations should be carried out in an environment equivalent to EU GMP grade A.

(g)   The transfer of materials into and out of the controlled workspace is a critical aspect of the isolator operation. Transfer devices should be designed such that they do not compromise the grade A working zone during the transfer of components. Commissioning studies should include tests to confirm that contaminants will not pass into the critical zone. A fully validated transfer procedure should be written and implemented (see Appendix 2, section A2.4).

(h)   The size and shape of the transfer device should be sufficient to allow all necessary materials and equipment to be passed through.

(i)   The controlled workspace of isolators that are used for the preparation of hazardous pharmaceuticals, e.g. cytotoxic drugs and radiopharmaceuticals, should operate at a negative pressure with respect to the background environment or be designed in such a way as to maximise operator protection as well as maintaining an appropriate level of product protection. Ideally these isolators should exhaust to the outside environment, with appropriate safeguards.

(j)   Dedicated clothing should be worn by isolator operators. The clothing worn should be appropriate to the background environment of the isolators.

(k)   There should be a designated changing room.

(l)   The operational characteristics of the isolator should be confirmed following any planned and unplanned maintenance.

7

Documentation

7.1   Documentation – general issues

(a)   A comprehensive documentation system should be prepared and approved in conjunction with the quality assurance officer.

(b)   All documents should be clear and detailed. Within any one unit, worksheets and labels should have a standardised style and presentation.

(c)   All documents should be regularly reviewed at defined intervals. Superseded documents should be clearly identified as such and should be retained for a sufficient period to satisfy legislative requirements.

7.2   Standard operating procedures

Standard operating procedures should be written in the imperative and should include the following:

- control of documentation systems
- receipt of orders, including prescription verification and transcription
- purchasing, receipt and storage of components
- cleaning, disinfection and sanitation processes
- entering and exiting from clean areas, including the correct use of protective clothing
- environmental monitoring (both physical and microbiological) of the clean rooms, laminar flow cabinets and isolators
- use of any equipment required for preparation, including cleaning and calibration instructions where appropriate
- product preparation, checking and release
- process validation, including media fills
- staff training, including broth transfer trials and formal skills assessment
- actions to be taken when failures are identified by the monitoring

systems, e.g. process simulations or operator validation tests, environmental monitoring and sterility tests

- storage and distribution
- product complaints and recalls, and handling of defective products (including, where appropriate, a defect log).

7.3   Worksheets

(a)   Individual worksheets reproduced from a suitably approved master format should be used. The worksheet should be sufficiently detailed to allow the traceability of starting materials and components to establish an audit trail for the product.

Completed worksheets should be retained for a sufficient period to satisfy legislative requirements.

(b)   Worksheets will vary for each unit and should be designed to minimise the possibility of transcription errors. They should include:

- the name and/or formula of products
- a unique number to identify the product
- a written protocol for routinely prepared products
- suppliers and batch numbers of medicinal ingredients
- suppliers and batch numbers of sterile components used to prepare the product, where appropriate
- date of preparation
- expiry date and time (if applicable) of product
- the signature or initials of staff carrying out preparation and checking procedures
- the signature or initials of the authorised pharmacist supervising the preparation process
- the signature or initials of the authorised pharmacist releasing the product
- a label reconciliation procedure for all labels
- a record of the label on the product
- the patient's name (where applicable)
- a comments section for recording any unusual occurrences or observations.

7.4   Records and reports

(a)   Operation, cleaning, maintenance and fault logs should be kept for all facilities and equipment. All planned preventative maintenance and breakdown maintenance should be recorded for key equipment and facilities.

(b)   A quality exception report should be available for all products made outside the standard operational procedures. Where deviations from specifications occur, written procedures should exist describing measures taken to ensure that the final product is satisfactory.

(c)   A record should be maintained of errors and near-misses and of investigations undertaken.

7.5   Computers

When computers are used for the calculation of product formulae and subsequent generation of labels and documentation, programs should be validated to ensure accuracy (see Appendix 2, section A2.7). Access to the computer should be restricted to authorised personnel by the use of passwords or another security system.

7.6   Labels

Labels must comply with all statutory and professional requirements, and should include the following information:

- approved name of medicine
- quantity and strength
- vehicle containing the drug
- final volume
- route of administration
- preparation date
- expiry date and time (if applicable)
- batch number
- appropriate cautionary notices
- storage requirements
- name of patient, patient's location
- name and address of pharmacy.

8

Personnel, training and competency assessment

8.1 Personnel and training – general issues

(a) Any aseptic preparation service must be managed by a responsible pharmacist who has current practical and theoretical experience in aseptic preparation and/or manufacture. He/she should be knowledgeable in all aspects of aseptic preparation, including the following areas:

- GMP as defined by the EU guide[10]
- formulation
- validation
- aseptic processing
- quality assurance
- quality control.

The responsible pharmacist must be assured that the facilities and systems in place are capable on a day-to-day basis of providing an adequate quality service able to meet the needs of patients.

(b) Any pharmacist called on to deputise for the responsible pharmacist should have the necessary level of training and knowledge, and be clear about the limits of his/her authority and responsibility.

(c) Day-to-day supervision of the service provided can be delegated to an authorised pharmacist provided that this pharmacist is given clear and precise training in both his/her duties and the limits of authority and responsibility.

8.2 Training

(a) Before undertaking aseptic work, all staff should be trained to an agreed level, which should be assessed. In particular, radiopharmacy staff must achieve 'adequate training' as defined in *The Ionising Radiation (Medical Exposure) Regulations*.[39]

All staff should receive training that will provide them with:

- an appropriate knowledge of GMP
- a knowledge of local practices, including health and safety
- competence in the necessary aseptic skills
- a knowledge of pharmaceutical microbiology
- a working knowledge of the department, products and services provided.

(b)   A written training programme to provide the above should be available and completion of this training should be documented. A system for the evaluation of the training programme, paying particular attention to practical skills, should be implemented (see Appendix 2, section A2.5).

8.3   Competency assessment

(a)   Regular reassessment of the competency of each member of staff should be undertaken, and revision or retraining provided where necessary.

(b)   A key element of operator competency is regular assessment of aseptic technique using broth. The recommended procedure is given in Appendix 2, section A2.2. This should be complemented by regular observation of aseptic technique to ensure that the operator can prepare dosage units precisely and safely.

(c)   Where a suitably trained member of staff has been absent from the aseptic operation for more than 6 months, the responsible pharmacist should assure him/herself as to the competence of that member of staff before allowing him/her to resume aseptic preparation.

(d)   There should be a commitment to a programme of ongoing training for all staff.

8.4   Staff hygiene

(a)   Standards of hygiene are of critical importance in aseptic processing.

(b)   Staff must be required to report infections and skin lesions.

(c)   Wrist watches and jewellery other than a simple wedding ring should
not be worn. Cosmetics should not be worn in clean areas.

8.5   Other personnel

Staff, service engineers and visitors not involved in the aseptic preparation process should observe the rules on clothing applicable for the
area. (A simplified training procedure on the elements of GMP for personnel entering the clean room facility, e.g. engineers and cleaning
staff, should also be available.)

9

Aseptic processing

(a) All manipulative steps in the aseptic process, from the raw material to the finished product, should be controlled by comprehensive standard operating procedures to ensure that the output of the process is a sterile product of the requisite quality.

(b) The key elements of the aseptic process include:
- maintaining the integrity of the aseptic processing area, and care of the workstation and its environment
- handling and preparation of starting materials, especially disinfection processes
- entry of materials into the processing area
- standard aseptic processing techniques, including 'no-touch' of critical surfaces, correct positioning of materials within laminar flow cabinets and the use of specific pieces of equipment
- segregation and flow of materials to ensure no inadvertent cross-contamination or muddling of prescriptions
- removal of product and waste materials from the processing area.

(c) All aseptic processing must be carried out and supervised by competent staff.

(d) Staff should be fully conversant with all relevant standard operating procedures before commencing work in the department. Regular updating of staff on the procedures should be undertaken, documented and the extent of knowledge assessed.

(e) No deviation should be allowed from the standard operating procedures. Should unusual circumstances necessitate deviation, this should be sanctioned by an appropriately experienced senior member of staff and fully documented.

(f) All staff working in aseptic processing should be made fully aware of the potential consequences of any deviation from the validated procedures, both to the integrity of the product and to the intended recipient. Regular reminders of the critical nature of the process should be provided.

(g)   Standard operating procedures should be written and implemented for all equipment used for aseptic processing. Where appropriate, equipment should be regularly calibrated and the accuracy of volume-measuring devices validated.

10

Monitoring

10.1 Monitoring – general issues

Regular monitoring of the environment, process and finished product is an essential part of the quality assurance of all aseptically prepared products. Standards and guidelines are available for many of the physical and microbiological aspects.[6, 10, 36–38, 40–44] The responsible pharmacist and senior staff should refer to and have an understanding of these documents, with particular emphasis on the sections relating to aseptic processing.

Particular importance should be attached to obtaining meaningful results, monitoring trends and setting 'in-house' standards and action limits. Information should be actively and knowledgeably assessed and not merely filed for record purposes.

10.2 Monitoring of the environment and clean-air devices

(a) Senior personnel within the aseptic preparation department must have an understanding of clean room and device technology together with a thorough knowledge of all the particular design features in their department, e.g. ventilation systems, position and grade of HEPA filters, type of workstation, isolator design, etc.

(b) All areas associated with the aseptic preparation process should be assessed by the quality assurance officer for compliance with the appropriate standards on commissioning, following maintenance procedures and routinely at an agreed frequency.

A written report of the test data indicating the significance of the results and recommended action must be brought to the attention of all relevant staff and full records kept on file for future reference.

10.2.1 Programme of monitoring

Each unit should have a programme of sessional, daily, weekly, monthly, quarterly and annual testing, with all results documented and retained for inspection. A recommended frequency of monitoring is shown for guidance in Tables 10.1 and 10.2. This should be considered to be a minimum requirement. The optimum frequency of testing will be a function of the individual unit and the activity within the unit. The programme should be such that it confirms that control of the environment within standards is maintained. It is not a substitute for the continual vigilance of operators in ensuring the correct functioning of all equipment.

Table 10.1 Microbiological monitoring programme

Test	Critical zone	Clean room suite
Finger dabs	Sessional	Not applicable
Settle plates	Sessional	Weekly
Surface sample	Weekly	Weekly
Active air sample	Three monthly	Three monthly

Table 10.2 Physical monitoring programme

Test	Critical zone	Clean room suite
Pressure differential between rooms	Not applicable	Monitor continuously, record daily
Pressure differential across HEPAs	Monitor continuously, record weekly	Monitor continuously, record three monthly
Particle counts	Three monthly	Three monthly
Air changes/hour, rooms	Not applicable	Three monthly
Air velocity, devices	Three monthly	Not applicable
HEPA filter integrity and leaks	Annual	Annual
Operator Protection Test BS5726	Annual	Not applicable
Isolator, glove integrity	Sessional	Not applicable
Isolator, leak test	Weekly	Not applicable
Isolator, alarm function	Weekly	Not applicable

10.2.2 Test limits for environmental monitoring

When undertaking microbiological testing, because of the imprecision of the methods compared to chemical and physical analysis and the expected low levels of contamination, the data require most careful analysis. Warning levels should be established well within the guideline limits provided in Tables 10.3 and 10.4. Exceeding the warning levels on isolated occasions may not require more action than examination of the control systems. However, the frequency of exceeding the limit should be examined and should be low. If the frequency is high or shows an upward trend then action should be taken.

For pharmaceutical applications the major criteria on which the aseptic facilities are assessed should be the risk of microbiological contamination of the product. However, because of the imprecision and variability of the microbiological test methods it is sometimes more practical to demonstrate environmental control using physical data. Guideline limits for physical and microbiological data are given in Tables 10.3 and 10.4. These limits are based on EU GMP[10] requirements and ISO14644.[37]

Table 10.3 Environmental monitoring of controlled areas and devices: limits for physical tests.

Grade	Particle counts (maximum particles/m³)				Air changes (number per hour)	Air-flow velocity (m/s ±20%)	Operator protection factor	Pressure differential to adjacent low-class room (Pa)
	At rest		In operation					
	0.5 μm	5.0 μm	0.5 μm	5.0 μm				
A (device)	3 500	0	3 500	0	N/A	0.45 HLF 0.30 VLF	>10⁵ VLF BS5726	LFC N/A Isolator >15
B	3 500	0	350 000	20 000	>20	N/A	N/A	>10
C	350 000	2 000	3 500 000	20 000	>20	N/A	N/A	>10
D	3 500 000	20 000	Not defined		>10	N/A	N/A	>10

N/A = not applicable.
Note: It is important that the required clean-up time is achieved.[10]
HLF = horizontal laminar flow; VLF = vertical laminar flow.

Table 10.4 Environmental monitoring of controlled areas and devices: limits for microbiological tests in operation

Grade	Finger dabs (cfu/hand)	Settle plates (90 mm) (cfu/4 hours)	Contact plate diameter (cfu/55 mm)	Active air sample (cfu/m³)
A (device)	<1	<1	<1	<1
B	Not applicable	5	5	10
C	Not applicable	50	25	100
D	Not applicable	100	50	200

If settle plates are exposed for less than 4 hours, then the warning levels should be adjusted accordingly. Validated surface swabbing may be used as an alternative to contact plates.

10.2.3 Equipment used for monitoring

(a)   Equipment used in monitoring must be serviced at least annually, calibrated and the results documented.

(b)   Settle plates, etc. should not be contaminated prior to their introduction into the aseptic processing environment. Ideally, overwrapped irradiated plates with certificates of analysis for each delivery should be used. The microbiological media used must be proven to be capable of supporting a broad spectrum of bacterial and fungal growth.

(c)   Steps should be taken to ensure that surface sampling materials do not leave media residues.

10.3   Monitoring the aseptic preparation process

(a)   It is important that all staff, on commencing aseptic preparation, assure themselves that all equipment is functioning satisfactorily. Potential problems should be reported to senior staff. Relevant records should be kept as defined in local procedures.

(b)   When the unit is in use the critical zone of the controlled workspace should be monitored on a sessional basis. This may be achieved by the exposure of settle plates, finger dabs of the gloved hand at the end of the work session and, if required, active air sampling.

(c)   Process validation using broth to simulate the aseptic procedure should be performed initially and subsequently on a regular basis.

10.4 Monitoring of finished products

(a)   There should be a planned programme of physical, chemical and microbiological analysis of the finished product as appropriate.

(b)   Samples may be obtained from:

- unused products
- extra specially prepared samples
- an in-process sample taken at the end of the compounding procedure before the final seals are in place and before removal from the critical zone.

(c)   Sampling of the final container after completion of preparation and prior to issue may be a threat to product integrity and is therefore not recommended.

(d)   The testing laboratory must be fully conversant with the technical background and requirements in aseptic preparation together with the validated methodology for analysing the products and samples. The responsible pharmacist should ensure that the testing laboratory has a comprehensive knowledge of pharmaceutical microbiology. An example of a technical agreement is given in Appendix 3.

10.5 Review and auditing

It is the responsibility of the chief pharmacist to ensure that quality assurance systems are regularly reviewed and that any off-site testing is regularly audited.

11

Cleaning

11.1 The facility

(a) The emphasis on providing the correct level of cleanliness is to ensure that the properly designed and maintained area is clean and dry. Dry dusting alone is not recommended. Wet or damp cleaning with effective detergents should be the method of choice. Depending on monitoring results, the use of a disinfectant may need to be considered. However, disinfection is difficult to achieve in an area with even small amounts of dirt.[45]

(b) Clean areas must be regularly cleaned and, where necessary, disinfected according to a written approved procedure. A log should be kept of the areas cleaned, indicating the agents used. This should be checked for completeness before filing.

(c) Any staff performing cleaning duties should have received documented training, including the relevant elements of GMP, and be assessed to be competent before being allowed to work alone.

(d) There should be continuity of cleaning staff with adequate suitably trained cover.

(e) The effectiveness of cleaning should be routinely demonstrated, at least weekly, by microbiological surface sampling, e.g. using contact plates or swabs.

(f) If results show an increase in microbiological contamination, the use of disinfection and/or an alternative disinfectant should be considered.

(g) Dedicated equipment should be used and stored to minimise microbiological contamination. Mopheads must be disposed of or resterilised after each cleaning session.

(h)   Cleaning and disinfecting agents should be free from viable micro-organisms. In-use dilutions should be freshly prepared for each cleaning session and should be periodically monitored for microbiological contamination before and after use.

(i)   Where disinfecting agents are used they should be approved by quality control.

11.2 The controlled workspace

(a)   Clean-air devices should be cleaned and disinfected before and after each working session with approved sterile agents.

(b)   The ability to sterilise isolators with a gaseous agent should be considered at the time of purchase.

        Note: Sterilisation is not a substitute for physical cleaning of the isolator.

(c)   The effectiveness of cleaning and disinfection should be routinely demonstrated, at least weekly, by microbiological surface sampling, e.g. using contact plates or swabs.

11.3 The transfer procedure

(a)   Surface disinfection prior to the introduction of items into hatches, both for conventional clean rooms and for isolators, is a vital step in preventing the ingress of contamination into critical areas. The process must have a written validated standard operating procedure (see Appendix 1). The contact time should be clearly stated, validated and maintained in practice.

(b)   Staff should wear gloves, which should be disinfected or sterilised prior to use, to transfer material into and out of an isolator.

(c)   Health and safety aspects must be considered for relevant disinfecting and sterilising agents, and also for dealing with spillages of chemicals and products, e.g. cytotoxics.

12

Starting materials, components and other consumables

12.1 Starting materials

(a)   Starting materials should ideally be sterile products with a product licence. Where unlicensed products are used, it is incumbent on the responsible pharmacist to ensure that the product is of appropriate quality by means of specifications, certificates of analysis or conformity, quality control tests or a combination of these.

        Unlicensed materials should always be obtained from a supplier with an appropriate manufacturer's licence.

        Non-sterile starting materials should not be used.

(b)   For unpreserved starting materials, the in-use shelf-life should be restricted to one working session (not exceeding 4 hours) during which the material remains in the critical zone. This may be modified if evidence is available to show compliance with the current *British Pharmacopoeia* (BP)[46] tests for preservative efficacy and sealability of the septum.

12.2 Components and other consumables

Components include:

- reconstitution devices
- syringes and needles
- the parts of filling systems in direct contact with the product
- transfer tubing
- final containers.

(a)   Components should ideally be purchased presterilised from the manufacturer. The product should be either CE marked or have a documented form of approval. It should be packaged in such a way that it can be passed into the aseptic environment without increasing the risk of product or environmental contamination.

(b)   Any filters used should be pre-assembled by the manufacturer and guaranteed sterile.

(c)   Local sterilisation of non-sterile components and equipment is acceptable provided that sterility is assured. Such sterilisation processes should be validated, appropriately monitored and meet all current standards.[47, 48] An audit trail should be available.

(d)   Filling systems, etc. should preferably not be modified, but if this is done it should be demonstrated that such modification does not jeopardise product sterility.

(e)   Sterile components should be stored so as to minimise any increase in the bioburden on the surface of the primary packaging.

(f)   Sterile components should not be used beyond one working session.

13

Product approval

(a) A formal recorded decision of approval should be taken by an authorised pharmacist before a preparation can be released.

(b) The authorised pharmacist should be suitably trained.

(c) The authorised pharmacist should not, other than in exceptional circumstances, be the person who prepared the product.

Note: It is recognised that circumstances can arise where the same person prepares and approves the product for use, e.g. residents working alone out of hours.

(d) There should be a written release procedure giving details of the role and responsibility of all the staff involved in the process.

(e) The authorised pharmacist should, before release:

- carry out a visual inspection of the product
- ensure that the product complies with the prescription and the appropriate specification, including labelling
- ensure that the product has been produced in accordance with the approved and validated operating procedures, and be aware of any quality exception reports
- be aware of recent microbiological and environmental results for the facilities
- ensure that the daily monitoring records for the unit are satisfactory, e.g. pressure differentials, cleaning
- be aware of recent retrospective testing results for products
- ensure that a reconciliation of empty and part-used containers of components and starting materials has been carried out.

(f) There should be a written procedure for dealing with preparations failing to meet the required standard. The investigation of these events should be fully documented and brought to the attention of the chief pharmacist.

14

Storage and distribution

(a) A close examination should be made of all stages between product approval and product use to ensure that the quality of the product is not compromised before its expiry.

(b) Products should be stored under refrigeration unless it would be detrimental to the product to do so.

(c) All refrigerators used for the storage of aseptic products within the pharmacy must be monitored to ensure compliance with the appropriate temperature range. This practice should also take place in the end-user department.

(d) For products where refrigeration is not appropriate, suitable storage conditions should be used to ensure no deterioration occurs.

(e) Due regard should be given to health and safety considerations relating to potential hazards posed by the products, both in storage and during distribution. All applicable regulations, e.g. *Control of Substances Hazardous to Health*[49] and transport regulations,[50–52] should be complied with. Labelling on transit containers of potentially hazardous products (e.g. cytotoxics) should include details of contacts and actions to be taken in an emergency.

(f) Distribution should be controlled and validated as rigorously as storage. Where necessary, the security of the cold chain should be assured. Transit containers should be of an appropriate defined specification and comply with any appropriate regulations.[50–52] The Trust's safety advisor should be able to provide additional information.

(g) Staff involved in storage and distribution should be aware of their responsibilities with regard to the integrity of the product. Training and assessment should be undertaken as appropriate and the results documented.

(h)   Records should be maintained of the destination of all products to ensure that effective recall can take place if necessary. Procedures for recall should be in place, and should be reviewed on a regular basis, to ensure the efficiency and timeliness of the process.

(i)   There should be a policy for the handling of returned or unused products.

15

Internal and external audit

(a) Audit involving all areas in which aseptic preparation takes place (including any satellites) should be undertaken on a regular planned basis[53] to monitor implementation and compliance with the guidance contained in this book.

(b) In addition to inspection of premises and equipment, detailed examination of documentation, production and quality control methods, validation, training and arrangements for dealing with complaints and recalls should also be undertaken as part of the audit programme.

(c) Observations made during audits should be clearly recorded along with any proposals for corrective measures. These corrective measures must be reviewed at the next audit or earlier if appropriate.

(d) The audit report should be submitted to the senior pharmacy manager responsible for the unit and a timescale agreed to remedy any deficiencies. Any deficiencies should be assessed in terms of risk to the quality of the product and a decision to cease activity made if necessary.

(e) There must be a regular programme of internal audit involving suitably experienced senior personnel.

(f) An external audit will also be carried out by the regional quality assurance specialist at least every 12 to 18 months.[8]

(g) Audits should include a review of the capacity planning within the unit (see Appendix 5).

Appendix 1

Specimen procedures for the transfer of materials
into the controlled workspace

The specimen procedures that follow are based on using a wiping and
spraying method of sanitation. The risks and benefits associated with
the stage at which primary packaging is removed should be carefully
considered. However, it is important that, whatever method is used,
the process should be validated and monitored for efficacy on a regular
basis (see Appendix 2, section A2.4).

The actual location of the disinfection stages will depend on the
design of the unit. The crucial factor is that two validated disinfection
stages should take place.

A1.1   Clean room and laminar flow cabinet facilities

(a)   Remove sterile wrapped items from all secondary packaging before
transfer from the storage area to the support room.

(b)   Wearing a fresh pair of disinfected disposable rubber or plastic gloves,
and using the disinfection process approved for use in the facility,
proceed as follows:

1.   Thoroughly disinfect all surfaces of the transfer hatch.
2.   Take a plastic or stainless steel tray and sanitise all its surfaces
carefully, ensuring that it is thoroughly wetted and being careful
not to miss the area by which the tray is being held. Place the tray
into the transfer hatch.
3.   Take one of the required items and sanitise all its surfaces, ensuring there is thorough and complete wetting, including where the
item is being held, and then place onto the previously treated
tray. It should be noted that paper labels, plastic vial caps and
visk rings are particularly difficult to disinfect.

4.   Repeat this procedure with every item, sanitising each one individually.

5.   Close the transfer hatch and leave all items for the validated contact time before moving to the next stage. This time period would not normally be less than 2 minutes.

(c)   Wearing sterile gloves, remove the items from the hatch into the clean room. Once the laminar flow cabinet has been prepared and sanitised, all items should once more be sanitised thoroughly using a sterile agent, ensuring that all surfaces are wetted. Place the items into the laminar flow cabinet, and again allow the validated contact time before taking any further action. Change or disinfect gloves before commencing work in the laminar flow cabinet.

A1.2   Pharmaceutical isolator facilities

(a)   Remove sterile wrapped items from all secondary packaging before transfer from the storage area to the support room.

(b)   Wearing a fresh pair of disinfected disposable rubber or plastic gloves, and using the disinfection process approved for use in the facility, proceed as follows:

1.   Thoroughly disinfect all surfaces of the transfer hatch.

2.   Take a plastic or stainless steel tray and sanitise all its surfaces carefully, ensuring that it is thoroughly wetted and being careful not to miss the area by which the tray is being held, or take a sterile tray. Place the tray into the transfer hatch. (Depending on the procedure in use in the unit, the standard of the background environment and the type of isolator, the tray should be placed in the transfer device and disinfected components placed onto it or the tray should be placed adjacent to the transfer device and moved into it when all disinfected components are ready in the tray.)

3.   Take one of the required items and sanitise all its surfaces, ensuring that there is thorough and complete wetting, including where the item is being held, and then place onto the tray. It should be noted that paper labels, plastic vial caps and visk rings are particularly difficult to disinfect.

4.   Repeat with every item, sanitising each one individually.

5.   When all items have been disinfected and placed in the transfer

device, close the transfer device and leave for the validated contact time before moving to the next stage.

(c)   Once the controlled workspace of the isolator has been prepared and sanitised, items being transferred in from the transfer device should again be sanitised thoroughly using a sterile agent, ensuring all surfaces are wetted. Place the items into the controlled workspace and leave for the validated contact time before taking further action.

Notes

1.   The Health and Safety Executive occupational exposure limit (OEL) for isopropyl alcohol is lower than that for industrial methylated spirit, therefore industrial methylated spirit is considered less hazardous.
2.   In rooms with poor ventilation, large amounts of spraying could result in OELs being exceeded. Wiping may be a safer alternative.
3.   Non-sterile disinfectant solutions should not be taken into a grade A[10] environment.

Appendix 2

Validation of aseptic preparation procedures

The quality assurance of any preparation activity is reliant on the satisfactory validation of the procedures. Validation should demonstrate that the overall process will reproducibly provide a product that complies with its specification.

Products that are prepared aseptically in hospital units should be sterile and should contain the correct chemical constituents at a concentration that is within acceptable defined limits.

Aseptic preparation activities in hospital aseptic units are individual unit processes that in most cases have a batch size of one. Batch production of multiple units is possible but analytical data for any one product would not be representative of the batch. Under such circumstances, the quality assurance of the process and the validation of the procedures used within the aseptic unit are of paramount importance.

This appendix is intended to give guidance on the design of validation programmes for critical procedures and activities within aseptic preparation units. Validation in the context of this book is understood to be the demonstration that a procedure achieves its desired outcome. This may be different from the statistical validation programmes that are designed for batch manufacturing processes, but is appropriate for the aseptic preparation activities of hospital units.

A validation programme may be designed before the facility or equipment are used, or before the product is made. However, sometimes this prospective validation is not carried out and retrospective validation can be successfully performed by review of historical data.[54]

The following procedures are covered in this appendix:

A2.1   microbiological validation of the process
A2.2   microbiological validation of the operator

A2.3 product validation
A2.4 validation of the transfer of materials into and out of the controlled workspace
A2.5 validation of training
A2.6 validation of cleaning processes
A2.7 computer validation.

A2.1 Microbiological validation of the process

Objective

To demonstrate that the procedures used during aseptic preparation and the staff undertaking aseptic processes are capable of maintaining the sterility of the product.

Procedure

1. A process simulation is a validation procedure that challenges both the operator and the facilities. The test is intended to simulate routine aseptic operations, but uses microbiological media to produce broth-filled units that can then be tested for contamination.
2. Procedures and facilities will be different depending on the type of product being prepared. PN preparations, a centralised intravenous additive and cytotoxic preparation are fundamentally different activities and so an appropriate test should be devised for each. Each operation should be analysed and a sequence devised that reflects the most complex practice.
3. All new processes should be validated not less than three times initially. Following this initial validation, a continuous programme of process validation should be established for all staff who use the aseptic unit. This programme should take account of the work pattern of the staff.
4. Tryptone soya broth would normally be used for these studies. This may be of double strength to allow for dilution during the test. Alternative liquid culture media may be used but the ability of the media to support the growth of contaminants should be demonstrated.
5. Broth-filled units should be incubated at the designated temperature for 14 days. If the final container is part-filled, all sur-

faces should be in contact with the broth at some time during incubation. A pass result requires no growth in all containers following incubation.

6. There should be a clearly defined procedure on action to be taken following any positive results. This should focus initially on whether the facilities, processes or operator practices are the cause of the failure. Revalidation of the process may also be appropriate.

More details about process validation can be found in the Parenteral Drug Association monograph *Validation of Aseptic Filling for Solution Drug Products*[41] and the Parenteral Society monograph *The Use of Process Simulation Tests in the Evaluation of Processes for the Manufacture of Sterile Products*.[55]

A2.2 Microbiological validation of the operator

Objective

To demonstrate that the aseptic technique of the operator undertaking aseptic processes is capable of maintaining the sterility of the product. Use of this universal operator validation test will allow for benchmarking comparisons between aseptic units and data analysis on a wider basis.

UNIVERSAL OPERATOR VALIDATION TEST

Introduction

(a) All aseptic manipulations can be broken down into a number of key techniques:

- withdrawing solution from an infusion bag
- withdrawing solution from a vial
- addition of solution to an infusion bag
- addition of solution to a vial
- withdrawing of a solution from an ampoule.

(b) All operators need to demonstrate competency in these techniques in order that they may prepare dosage units safely.

(c)   Staff should initially carry out a number of operator validation tests as part of their training programme. This number should be decided locally but would not normally be less than three. Following this initial validation a continuing programme of staff validation should be established for all staff who use the aseptic unit. This programme should take account of the work pattern of the staff.

Equipment

1 × 50 mL single-strength tryptone soya broth vial
3 × sterile glass vials 20 mL, labelled A, B and C.
1 × 100 mL single-strength tryptone soya broth infusion bag
1 × 10 mL ampoule single-strength tryptone soya broth
22 × 5 mL syringe
4 × syringe caps/blind hubs
Needles and other equipment (as per local procedure)
Departmental sanitisation materials (alcohol wipes and sprays)
4 tryptone soya settle plates (cabinet, room, finger dabs)

Note: All media used in this test should have been subjected to an appropriate test for sterility.

Procedure

Detailed worksheets for this procedure can be found on the National CIVAS Group website www.civas.co.uk. A schematic representation of the procedure outlined below is shown in Figure A2.1 (on p. 68).

1.   Follow local procedure for first-stage decontamination of materials into the clean room or isolator hatch, then second-stage transfer into the environment in which the validation procedure will be performed.
2.   Set out the equipment within the workstation.
3.   Ensure that settle plates are exposed in the room where the broth transfer is being performed and in the workstation.
4.   Wipe the additives port of the bag of single-strength broth using a sterile alcohol impregnated wipe. Using a 5 mL syringe remove 5 mL of broth from the bag. Cap the syringe.
5.   Using a new syringe and needle each time repeat step 4 a further four times, removing a total of 25 mL from the bag into five 5 mL syringes. Cap each syringe.

6. Wipe the top of the vial of single-strength broth with a sterile alcohol wipe. Using a 5 mL syringe remove 5 mL of broth from the vial and add it to the bag of broth.
7. Using a new syringe and needle each time repeat step 6 a further four times, transferring a total of 25 mL of broth from the vial to the bag.
8. Open the ampoule of single-strength broth and using a 5 mL syringe and needle remove 5 mL of broth. Place this in empty sterile vial A.
9. From the bag of single-strength broth remove 5 mL of broth, using a new 5 mL syringe, and place it in vial A.
10. Using new syringes and needles repeat steps 8 and 9 twice. A total of 20 mL of broth will now be in vial A.
11. Using a new 5 mL syringe remove 5 mL of broth from vial A and place it in vial B.
12. Using a new syringe repeat step 11. Vials A and B now both contain 10 mL of broth.
13. Using a new syringe and needle withdraw 5 mL of broth from vial B and place it in vial C. Vials B and C now contain 5 mL of broth.
14. Perform finger dabs according to local procedures.
15. Change gloves and proceed to clean down the workstation following local procedure.
16. Label the bag, the 50 mL vial, the syringes and vials A, B and C with the following details: name, date, room where validation performed. Also label the settle plates and finger dab plates.
17. Complete the details on the validation results form (see Form A2.1).
18. The bag, vials, syringes and plates should be incubated at 30–35°C for 14 days. They should be inspected daily (week-ends/bank holidays excepted).

Note: A positive control should be performed annually on the raw materials and consumables containing broth to demonstrate their ability to support the growth of organisms potentially present in the environment where the test is performed.

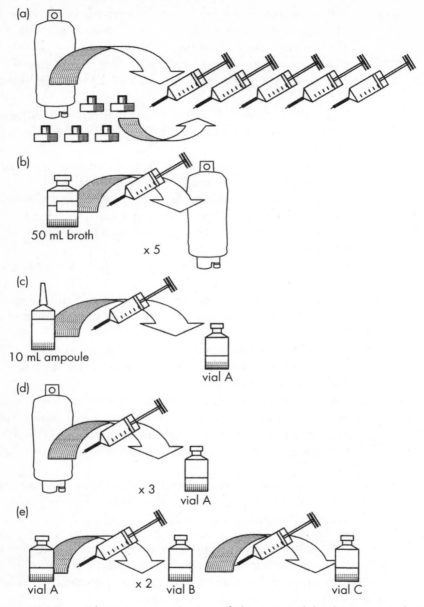

Figure A2.1 Schematic representation of the universal broth test procedure. (a) Transfer from bag to syringes: fill 5 × 5 mL syringes and cap. (b) Transfer from vial to bag: fill 5 × 5 mL syringes and add to bag. (c) Transfer from ampoule to vial: fill 1 × 5 mL syringe and add to vial A. (d) Transfer from bag to vial: fill 3 × 5 mL syringes and add to vial A. (e) Transfer from vial to vial: fill 2 × 5 mL syringes from vial A and add to vial B, and then fill 1 × 5 mL syringe from vial B and add to vial C.

| Results Form |

Operator name		Unit*		Date		Batch No.*	

*Where applicable

1. Environment of test

Section in pharmacy where test performed e.g. CIVAS / TPN / CYTOs	Workstation type (critical zone) e.g. horizontal or vertical LAFC, isolator	Test supervisor

2. Details of tryptone soya broth

Manufacturer of broth	Batch no.	Expiry date	Operator	Checker (where applicable)

3. Details of incubation

Incubator type and identifier	Incubation details from the chart recorder, e.g. 32 ± 2°C for 14 days	Incubation supervisor

Form A2.1 continues over

4. Results

4.1 Inspect daily: + for turbidity; − for clear; w/e for plates
not read at weekends

Item	Day														Pass or
	1	2	3	4	5	6	7	8	9	10	11	12	13	14	fail
Syringe 1															
Syringe 2															
Syringe 3															
Syringe 4															
Syringe 5															
Vial A															
Vial B															
Vial C															
Large vial															
Minibag															

4.2 Inspect plates at the end of the incubation period

	Results	Pass or fail
Room plate*		
Work plate*		
Left hand		
Right hand		

*Contamination on these plates may indicate an environmental problem rather than an operator problem and appropriate consideration should be taken of this in resultant action.

5. Release

Operator passes/fails test

Signature:_____ Date:_____

The presence of any turbidity in the vials, bags or syringes may indicate a fail. Presence of microbial contamination should be confirmed by appropriate microscopy or by subculturing and subsequent microbiological identification of the contaminating organism.

If growth occurs in the broth transfer test, the operator's authorisation to prepare aseptic products will be reviewed and may need to be suspended as specified in local procedures.

A2.3   Product validation

Objective

To confirm that the processes used will reproducibly produce a product containing the correct constituents at a concentration that is within acceptable limits and that the chemical and microbiological integrity of the product is maintained throughout its designated shelf-life.

Procedure

1. The stability of the product up to and during the time of administration should be proven and is a prerequisite for validation of the composition of the finished product.
2. The container of the finished product must be capable of maintaining its integrity, in respect of microbial and chemical contamination, up to the point of use. It is important that containers are purchased to a recognised standard in order to maintain a consistent design and quality, and it must be remembered that certain containers, e.g. disposable plastic syringes, are not designed for prolonged storage of pharmaceuticals. Validation of the integrity of the container may be carried out by filling the various types of container with sterile media. The containers are then stored at a temperature that promotes microbial growth, e.g. 30–35°C, under a variety of conditions that simulate the challenges of storage and transport. The outside of the container may be positively challenged by immersion in media containing a microbial culture. Any subsequent growth is noted. All containers should prevent the ingress of micro-organisms.
3. The documentation should include a recorded check that the correct ingredients have been used. Validation should confirm that this process is effective. Validation of the constituents of the product is achieved by carrying out a schedule of chemical or other appropriate analyses of the finished product that focuses on those components of most concern.
4. Validation of the microbiological quality of the product is achieved by carrying out a schedule of microbiological analysis of the finished product.
5. The results of the microbiological analysis of the product will probably only be known in retrospect. The microbiological

analysis of the finished product should not be confused with the *British Pharmacopoeia*[46] sterility test since the requirements for volume taken, number of containers and the ability to carry out a retest cannot generally be met. Any growth should be investigated. Comparison may be made between different compounding units as part of an external quality control scheme.

6. The number and frequency of samples to be analysed, both chemically and microbiologically, is at the discretion of the individual unit. Particular attention should be paid to new procedures and automated processes.

A2.4 Validation of the transfer of materials into and out of the controlled workspace

Objective

To demonstrate that the procedure used for the transfer of materials provides components and materials with surfaces that are free from viable organisms.

Procedure

1. Validation may be carried out either by using contact plates or by swabbing a specified area, e.g. 10 cm × 10 cm with a swab moistened with a suitable wetting solution.
2. The transfer of all types of container, e.g. bag, bottle, syringe, likely to be introduced into the controlled workspace must be validated.
3. Materials should be tested (using either swabs or contact plates) immediately prior to disinfection, i.e. at zero time. To validate the test procedure growth must be shown at this stage.
4. The materials should be transferred into the controlled workspace using the routine procedure, e.g. spraying, wiping.
5. After the designated contact time (timed with a stopwatch), sampling of all containers should be repeated on an equally sized area not previously tested. To validate the process there should be no growth for any sample.
6. A negative control (an unexposed contact plate or swab) can show that false positive contamination has not occurred.
7. A positive control (performed by swabbing, for example, an operator's ungloved hand or by using a contact plate on a known

'dirty' area) is also useful to demonstrate that the medium can support growth.

8. The validation process must be successfully repeated when the transfer procedure is modified in any way. The validation exercise should be repeated on a regular basis even if the procedure remains the same.

A2.5 Validation of training

Objective

To confirm that all staff have a satisfactory level of knowledge and competency for the duties they are required to undertake.

Procedure

Effective training is a critical part of the quality assurance of aseptic products. It is important that both the training programme and the impact on the trainee are effective.

1. The training programme should be fully documented and con-structed in a fashion that enables outcomes to be stated in terms of competencies, which are measurable.

2. The training programme should be validated by:
   (i) auditing the content by comparison with the appropriate elements of GMP
   (ii) checking that all necessary elements of the practical aspects of aseptic processing are incorporated within the pro-gramme (see the references for relevant source documents)
   (iii) ensuring that the documentation of training undertaken is comprehensive, including records of experience and compe-tency
   (iv) a review by an experienced trainer (not necessarily involved in the aseptic service) to ensure that all appropriate steps for effective training are incorporated and that adequate records are maintained.

3. The training process should be validated by performing compe-tency checks on trainees before training, after training and after a further time interval to ensure that learning does take place and is retained. Competency can be assessed by:

(i)   verbal questioning
(ii) written questionnaire
(iii) supervisor observation
(iv) simulation of the activity.

4. Competency should be reassessed on a regular basis and deficiencies rectified by additional training.

5. Periodic overview of the competency checks by an independent experienced operator may also be useful.

A2.6 Validation of cleaning processes

Objective

To confirm that chemical, microbiological and other contaminants are removed or inactivated during the cleaning process.

Procedure

1. For both microbiological and chemical validation of cleaning, sampling should be carried out before the cleaning process (to reflect the worst case) and afterwards to demonstrate the efficiency of the process. This is particularly important in clean areas and where hazardous materials, e.g. antibiotics, cytotoxic agents and radiopharmaceuticals, are involved. The use of dye may help to indicate whether or not cleaning procedures are adequate.

2. A programme detailing the numbers and positions of sites to be tested, along with the frequency of testing, should be decided locally depending on factors such as workload in the unit, rotation and experience of staff, and operator safety.

3. Swabs over specified areas are recommended for detecting chemical contamination, and either swabs or contact plates may be used for the microbiological validation of cleaning. Contact plates can be useful for the validation of cleaning processes relating to clean-room garments.

4. Although surfaces should not be deliberately contaminated, a positive control (e.g. swabbing an operator's hand or using a contact plate on a dirty area) can be useful to demonstrate that growth is supported. A negative control (where a swab is merely moistened with test vehicle or a contact plate is not exposed) may

also be used to demonstrate that the validation process does not give false positive results.

5. The standard operating procedure for the validation of cleaning processes should include subsequent action, e.g. detailed examination of the cleaning procedure itself, if any residual contamination is detected.

6. All cleaning processes and their validation should be thoroughly documented.

7. The retrospective results of cleaning validation should be considered when determining batch approval.

8. Specific guidance on testing for chemical surface contamination using simple low-cost methods is available in an accompanying regional quality control document.[56] Methods for many common antibiotics and cytotoxic agents are included.

A2.7 Computer validation

Objective

To confirm that computer hardware and software systems perform to the requisite standards, delivering an output that is accurate and free of errors.

Procedure

1. Successful validation requires the careful selection of a computer system, with consideration given to the possible benefits of computerisation against the costs and effort involved in setting up and validating any system.

2. Computerised systems must ensure that quality system standards are maintained or improved over any manual system that they replace.

3. A user requirement specification should be prepared prior to the purchase of any computerised system, defining the requirements against which any system is to be validated.

4. The requirement for backup systems and contingency plans for computer system failure should be included in the user requirement specification.

5. Suppliers should be required to provide evidence that they have developed any software against recognised guidelines and standards, including:
   (i) *The TickIT Guide ISO9002*[57]
   (ii) IEEE standards[58, 59]
   (iii) *Guide to Good Automated Manufacturing Practice (GAMP).*[60]

6. A workflow and risk analysis should be completed to identify system limitations and weaknesses, and requirements for supporting systems and procedures.

7. All documentation relating to the computerised system should be logged.

8. All computer systems used in conjunction with aseptic processing should be secure. Different levels of password access should be available to different users of the system. Demonstrable restricted high-level password access should be present so that critical data can be protected. An audit trail should be present, recording all attempts at access to the system (successful or not).

9. Where computers are used solely for documentation generation, and no computation or calculation is undertaken by the computer program, then no further validation is necessary, provided checks are made of the documentation generated against an approved master document every time.

10. Where a computer system holds critical data (e.g. the electrolyte content of a solution used for preparation of TPN solutions), the integrity of this data should be checked as part of the initial validation of the system.

11. Where a computer system is used to control an automated piece of equipment (e.g. a parenteral nutrition compounder), the validation processes defined in the GAMP[60] guide should be followed. Key to this are:
    (i) installation qualification
    (ii) operational qualification
    (iii) performance qualification.

12. If the computerised system is replacing a manual process, operation of the two systems in parallel for an appropriate period, with comparison of the output of the two systems, should constitute part of the validation process.

13. When a new computerised system is introduced it should not be used for the preparation of products that will be administered to patients until a validation report has been completed and the system authorised for use by the quality assurance officer.

14. Where critical data on which subsequent calculation is based (e.g. a patient's weight for paediatric PN) is entered manually, a check should be performed of this critical data entry, whether electronically or by a second operator. The integrity of this checking procedure should form part of the procedures for validation of the system of working.

15. Procedures should be established to revalidate the system after any of the following:
    (i)   system malfunction (e.g. where data has become corrupted or lost)
    (ii)   new version of software installed (new or greatly enhanced functionality)
    (iii) new software release (minor developments in the software plus patches developed to overcome reported problems).

16. Where a networking system is used to link a number of terminals together, the validation of the system should take into account the effect of the network on the operation of the system. When changes to the network are made consideration should be given as to the degree of revalidation required.

17. Comprehensive records should be retained of all validation programmes and the results obtained. Hard copies should be retained of all system release notes and software alerts issued by the software supplier.

18. Staff training programmes for the use of computerised systems should be documented and training records kept.

Appendix 3

Model technical agreement for the supply of
microbiological services to the pharmacy aseptic unit
by the microbiological service

This agreement is made between the [name] NHS Trust, the Pharmacy Aseptic Unit (PAU) (the contract giver/purchaser) and the Microbiology Service Provider (MSP) (the contract acceptor), for:

- the supply of media
- the provision of microbiological testing procedures
- advice by the microbiology department.

Services will be provided on an ongoing annual basis with a review of workload and quality of service made at renewal. Details of the annual review will be provided to both the contract giver and contract acceptor.

- The provision of media will be as stated in section A.
- The microbiological testing procedures are as in section B.
- Section C outlines the frequency of samples provided.
- Provision of advice will be as in section D.
- Arrangements for extra work or special investigations are in section E.
- Inspection and audit work will be carried out as in section F.

Section A

Media

The MSP will supply an agreed range of media. For example:

Approximately [number] tryptone soya agar plates each week
Approximately [number] tryptone soya agar contact plates each week

The MSP may purchase plates or pour them. Plates will be provided to an agreed timetable. Transport arrangements will be in place for plates to be delivered promptly. For purchased plates, the packaging (e.g. double or triple wrapped) should be specified, as well as the fertility.

For poured plates, the MSP will provide:

- an audit trail for their empty petri dish suppliers to show that dishes used are sterile
- batch preparation to set formulae, with documentation completed at time of preparation allowing for checking of weights and volumes, and providing traceability for the batch
- media that have been fertility tested for four organisms on each batch: *Staphylococcus aureus*, *Bacillus* sp., *Escherichia coli* and *Candida albicans*. Reference strains will be used. The MSP will use a standard operating procedure acceptable to the PAU for fertility testing
- plates poured in clean conditions with every effort made to prevent contamination. All plates will be gamma irradiated to a minimum dose level of [units], according to a standard operating procedure, to ensure that the batch is not contaminated
- plates stored between preparation and dispatch in conditions that will minimise the risk of opportunistic contamination.

Section B

Microbiological methods

All plates and media submitted by the PAU will be incubated as soon as possible and at least within an agreed maximum period of receipt. Incubation will take place under defined conditions (temperature and duration). For example:

> *Plates will be incubated at ..., etc.*
> *Broth-filled containers will be incubated at ..., etc.*
> *For liquid samples, a membrane filtration method will be used according to a standard operating procedure. Incubation will be at ..., etc.*

Reporting of results will be to an agreed specification. For example:

> *For settle plates and contact plates, results will be read as the number of organisms per plate. For broth-filled containers, the*

results will be read as positive or negative growth. Where necessary, serial dilutions may need to be made using a suitable medium to enable accurate colony counts to take place. For liquid samples, results will be expressed as the number of organisms per unit volume.

For contact plates, settle plates and finger dabs in critical zones, and validation of alcohol and other liquids, the species of micro-organism will be identified. Morphological characteristics and simple testing methods, e.g. gram stain, will be used. Standard operating procedures will be used. Identification may also be required in other situations when limits are exceeded.

Results will be entered on the MSP's computer system and reported to the PAU in hard-copy format within an agreed timescale. Results will be dispatched with the next mail collection.

It is the responsibility of the MSP to maintain their incubating equipment to assure both parties that it performs to specification. This includes arranging for the chart recorder for the incubation facilities to be independently calibrated on at least an annual basis against a traceable standard.

Section C

Sampling frequency and details should be specified. An example is given in Table A3.1 on p. 82.

Section D

Advice

• The PAU will inform the MSP immediately of any significant changes to work schedules that will affect the routine service provided by the MSP.

• The MSP will inform the PAU immediately if there is an untoward incident that will prevent them providing their normal service to the PAU.

• The MSP will inform the PAU if it makes changes to its standard operating procedures that will affect the testing carried out for the PAU.

• The PAU will negotiate with the MSP to adjust services during bank holiday periods.

Table A3.1 An example of a record of sampling fequency

Frequency	Procedure	Numbers*	Microbiology procedure
Sessional	In-use settle plates – workstation	–	Number of organisms per plate Species of organism where appropriate
Sessional	Finger dabs – gloves in isolators	–	Number and species of organisms per plate Species of organism where appropriate
Weekly	Settle plates – room	–	Number of organisms per plate
Weekly	Water samples	–	Number of organisms per mL
Weekly	Contact plates – workstation surfaces	–	Number and species of organisms per plate
Monthly	Industrial methylated spirit validation	–	Number and species of organisms
Monthly	Broth transfer – personal	–	Positive or negative growth
Three monthly	Plates (active air sampling) for aseptic rooms	–	Number and species of organisms per plate
Three monthly	Plates (active air sampling) for cabinets	–	Number and species of organisms per plate
Three monthly	PN broth transfer	–	Positive or negative growth

*Entries in this column will depend on the units used.

- The MSP will provide an appropriate level of advice to the PAU in the event of unusual or out-of-specification results, untoward events or result trends.
- The MSP will ensure that advice is only provided by staff fully trained in pharmaceutical microbiology and the quality assurance of the aseptic preparation of medicines.
- Both departments will make arrangements as appropriate for new or existing staff to visit each other's department for induction and/or training purposes.

Section E

Extra work and special investigations

These will arise as a result of either an untoward event or as part of a planned programme, e.g. the commissioning of new equipment or facilities, or validation of a new processing method.

For planned work, the PAU will inform the MSP at an early stage. Negotiations will then take place to define requirements and arrange the most appropriate way to provide them.

For unplanned work, the same arrangements will take place but on an accelerated timescale.

A record of extra work will be kept by the MSP to be reviewed as part of the annual review process for this technical agreement. Workload variations, for example of $\pm 5\%$, should be allowed for within the contract.

Section F

Inspection and audit

It will be incumbent on the responsible pharmacist at the PAU to inspect the service being provided by the MSP to assure him/herself that the conditions of this agreement are being complied with. The responsible pharmacist will have the right to visit at any time, subject to convenience and confidentiality.

A formal audit will take place on an annual basis, at a time and date mutually agreed with the manager of the MSP. Any concerns will be discussed.

The report from this inspection will be reviewed as part of the renewal process.

The PAU will inform the MSP if, as part of their external audit, a body outside the Trust wishes to review the service provided under this agreement. Arrangement will be made at a time that is convenient to the MSP.

The responsibility for initiating any changes recommended as part of an external audit will be that of the PAU.

Section G

Contract duration

The contract duration should be specified (e.g. 5-year rolling contract, reviewed annually) and a termination notice period agreed.

Signed on behalf of the pharmacy aseptic unit

.... Responsible pharmacist

.... Name

.... Date

Signed on behalf of the microbiology service provider

.... Manager

.... Name

.... Date

Appendix 4

Products for short-term use – maximum shelf-life
24 hours

There are no shelf-lives quoted in the Medicines Act 1968[5] legislation but product data sheets produced as a condition of the product licence currently recommend that reconstituted and/or diluted injections are used within 24 hours, subject to satisfactory chemical stability. This recommendation applies to products prepared in uncontrolled environments.

As discussed in Chapter 3 (and stated in *Executive Letter (96) 95*[7]), there is an increased risk of microbial contamination of products prepared in uncontrolled environments. There is also an increased risk of medication errors when preparing injections without pharmacy supervision.

Wherever possible, aseptic products prepared under pharmacy control should be prepared in accordance with the standards set down in this book. In some circumstances, however, this may not be possible for clinical or operational reasons although risk assessment shows that safety would be increased by some degree of pharmacy control where the alternative would be preparation in an uncontrolled situation. In these circumstances some of the standards may be modified as detailed in this appendix but the shelf-life of the product would then be restricted to 24 hours. The expectation is that the product should be used immediately or, if not, stored at 2–8°C.[29]

The following commentary highlights where there are differences from the text in the main body of this book.

Chapter 4 – Management

The unit may be remote from the main pharmacy and the management of the facility may be shared with clinical medical or nursing staff.

Chapter 5 – Formulation, stability and shelf-life

According to patients' clinical needs, any product may be required at any time, often at very short notice. This may mean that there is no validated method of preparation and there may be very little time to assess information on stability. The Summary of Product Characteristics (SPC) recommendations should be followed where available. In this case the shortest possible shelf-life consistent with the intended use of the product should be given and in no circumstances should a shelf-life of 24 hours be exceeded.

Chapter 6 – Facilities

Pharmaceutical isolators may be located in a background environment that may not achieve airborne particulate contamination levels for grade D but achieves the recommended limits for microbial contamination set down in Tables A4.1 and A4.2.

Laminar air-flow cabinets should always be operated in accordance with the standards in the main text even when they are used to prepare products for short-term use.

It may not be possible to measure or indicate the pressure differentials between rooms in some locations.

Chapter 7 – Documentation

There may be no master worksheet for some uncommon products. The content of the worksheet may reflect the immediacy of supply but should be sufficiently detailed to allow traceability of starting materials and to establish an audit trail for the product.

Chapter 10 – Monitoring

The frequency of monitoring will be dependent on the function and activity of the unit but may be less than the minimum requirements set down in the main text. Alternatively, in a busy unit monitoring may be more frequent than the minimum requirements in the main text.

There may be no limits for the non-viable particle counts of the background environment and the limits for microbial contamination will be as set down in Tables A4.1 and A4.2.

Table A4.1 Products for short-term use. Environmental monitoring: limits for physical tests

	Isolators	
	Controlled workspace	Room
Pressure differential	>15 Pa	Not applicable
Non-viable particle counts (particles/m³)		
>0.5 μm	3500	Not specified
>5 μm	0	
>10 μm	0	

Table A4.2 Products for short-term use. Environmental monitoring: guidance limits for microbiological tests

	Isolators	
	Controlled workspace	Room
Settle plates, 90 mm, 4 hours exposure	One per two plates	200
Surface sample (55 mm plate)	One per two plates	50
Active air samples (cfu/m³)	<1	500
Finger dabs (cfu/5 fingers)	1	Not specified

Microbiological limits are in operational state.

Chapter 13 – Product approval

Products may need to be released at very short notice for clinical reasons and there may be no validated method of preparation for some products. Also, there may not be time for the authorised pharmacist releasing the product to be aware of all monitoring records and retrospective testing results.

Validation

Microbiological validation of the process and of the operators must be as specified in the main text but product validation is not appropriate for products for short-term use (within 24 hours) if they are prepared in accordance with the instructions in the product data sheet.

Appendix 5

Capacity planning – technical services

Introduction

Given the increasing workload pressures on existing resources, particularly in aseptic services, the need for technical services to prepare their own formalised 'capacity plans' should be viewed as a key service objective. The MCA's Inspectorate have themselves increasingly highlighted this aspect recently. The following guidance was originally written for North Thames Region pharmacy production managers to be used as a basis for preparing their own more detailed local capacity plans.

Guidance notes

Capacity planning is a system used to assess:

- the volumes and types of workloads that need to be undertaken within given timeframes
- the resources (staff, facilities, equipment, etc.) necessary to meet these workloads
- the various strategies that could be adopted when available resources are inadequate.

Workload includes not only those direct production activities needed to make a product but also indirect activities ancillary to the production process, e.g. ordering, stock control, product testing and distribution, or necessary to maintain the infrastructure of the department, e.g. training, standard operating procedure/worksheet maintenance, administration, validation, audit, maintenance and monitoring, etc.

Capacity planning is required to ensure that:

- response and lead times remain within agreed limits
- quality and safety standards and standard operating procedures are not compromised
- excessive overtime is not worked by staff
- excessive pressure is not placed on staff
- errors and defective product rates do not increase.

Capacity planning should be considered at two levels:

1. medium to long term: 6/12+ monthly basis
2. acute: daily/weekly basis

Medium- to long-term planning

Key quantitative indicators that can be used to assess whether or not there have been sufficient resources available to meet workload over a period of time include:

- overtime worked
- response times, lead times and number of 'out-of-stocks'
- error rates, number of product defects and numbers of recorded deviations from standard operating procedures
- targets for 'indirect' activities (percentage met)
- numbers of complaints.

These indicators should be compared with previous monitoring periods and if deteriorating, the root cause should be established. For example, is the change due to:

- a shortfall in trained staff, e.g. vacancies, increased numbers of trainees, new or rotational staff, increased sickness levels, etc.?
- an increase in production throughput or complexity of product range?
- a shortage of space, equipment capacity or equipment failure?

If such factors are likely to continue into the next planning period, the following actions should be considered:

- introduce efficiency measures
- modify (skill mix) or increase staffing levels
- purchase additional or replacement equipment
- identify additional space
- reduce production volume.

Benchmarking[53] against other hospital units with a similar profile in terms of types of services, and the range and volume of products produced may provide useful information in determining the most appropriate action to take.

Assessing workload

The staff time required to prepare different types of product using different processing methods can vary significantly. For production units with a complex mix and high volume of products, assessing workload changes (and calculating the staffing resources required) could be made simpler if standard work units (reflecting 'activity' time) are assigned to each product category or task.

Assessing staffing

In order to assess the staffing resources required/available, their number, type and status must be identified:

Numbers	in work, in post, establishment
Type	assistant technical officers, medical technical officers, pharmacists, student technicians, preregistration pharmacists
Status	trainees, trained, accredited, permanent, rotational, new, agency

Actual or projected allowances should be made for the following:

- annual leave
- sickness, especially long-term sickness
- study leave
- down time (tea breaks, idle time, etc.)
- vacancies (number and period)
- maternity leave
- indirect activities (e.g. planned preventative maintenance, training, etc.)
- 'time out' to work on service/personal objectives.

Assessing facilities and equipment

It is important to identify any rate-limiting factors in terms of workspace, numbers and size or type of equipment in use, e.g. controlled workstations, sterilisers and space to inspect/check/label products.

Acute planning

Each day or week production sections should assess:

- direct production workload planned or anticipated (e.g. types of product, number of work units required)
- trained and accredited staff time available
- facilities and equipment available

and establish if any shortfall or surplus exists. As an aid to this assessment process it may be useful to prepare a capacity planning matrix that correlates for different categories of product the maximum number of doses/units that can be prepared in a given timeframe with the numbers of trained staff needed. If there is a shortfall in staff, facilities or equipment or too high a workload, predetermined strategies should be put into place. These might include one or more of the following:

- deferring doses or product not required the same day
- deferring indirect or other non-production activities not essential to be undertaken the same day
- transferring trained staff to areas of greatest need (e.g. higher risk products required the same day)
- using ready-made standard products or intermediates
- smoothing out workflow during the day or week by ordering or preparing in advance
- overtime
- staff working down a grade
- transferring work to another unit (internal or external)
- transferring lower risk, lower complexity, low-cost centralised intravenous additive doses back to wards. (This should be a last resort.)

References

1. Breckenridge A. *The Report of the Working Party on the Addition of Drugs to Intravenous Infusion Fluids (HC(76)9)*. (The Breckenridge Report) London: Department of Health and Social Security, 1976.

2. *The Quality Assurance of Aseptic Preparation Services*, 1st edn. Quality Control Sub-Committee of the Regional Pharmaceutical Officers Committee, Mersey Regional Health Authority, 1993.

3. Medicines Control Agency. *Guidance to the NHS on the Licensing Requirements of the Medicines Act 1968*. London: Medicines Control Agency, 1992.

4. Lee MG, ed. *The Quality Assurance of Aseptic Preparation Services*, 2nd edn. Liverpool: NHS Quality Control Committee, 1996.

5. The Medicines Act 1968. London: HMSO, 1968.

6. Farwell J. *Aseptic Dispensing for NHS Patients*. (The Farwell Report) London: Department of Health, 1995.

7. NHS Executive. *Executive Letter (96) 95: Aseptic Dispensing in NHS Hospitals*. London: Department of Health, 1996.

8. NHS Executive. *Executive Letter (97) 52: Aseptic Dispensing in NHS Hospitals*. London: Department of Health, 1997.

9. Lee MG, ed. *The Quality Assurance of Aseptic Preparation Services Supplement on Products for Short Term Use*. Liverpool: NHS Quality Control Committee, 1999.

10. Medicines Control Agency. *Rules and Guidance for Pharmaceutical Manufacturers and Distributors 1997*. London: HMSO, 1997.

11. NHS Executive. *The New NHS: Modern, Dependable*. London: Department of Health, 1997.

12. NHS Executive. *A First Class Service – Quality in the New NHS.* London: Department of Health, 1998.

13. NHS Executive. *Controls Assurance Standards.* NHS Executive, Feb 2000.

14. *High Efficiency Air Filters (HEPA and ULPA) Classifications, Performance Testing and Marking. BS EN 1822–1: 1998.* Milton Keynes: British Standards Institute, 1998.

15. Cousins DH, Upton DR. How to prevent IV drug errors. *Pharm Pract* 1997; 7: 310–312.

16. Sklar GE. Propofol and postoperative infections. *Ann Pharmacother* 1997; 31: 1521–1523.

17. Daily MK, Dickey JB, Packo KH. Endogenous *Candida endophthalmitis* after intravenous anaesthesia with propofol. *Arch Ophthalmol* 1991; 109: 1081–1084.

18. Bennett SN, McNeill MM, Bland LA, *et al.* Post operative infections traced to contamination of an intravenous anaesthetic, propofol. *N Engl J Med* 1995; 333: 147–154.

19. Kuehnert MJ, Webb RM, Jochinsen EM, *et al. Staphylococcus aureus* bloodstream infections among patients undergoing electroconvulsive therapy traced to breaks in infection control and possible extrinsic contamination by propofol. *Anaes Analg* 1997; 85: 420–425.

20. Ernot L, Thoren S, Sandell E. Studies on microbial contamination of infusion fluids arising from drug additions and administration. *Pharmaceutica Suecica* 1973; 10: 141–146.

21. Cos GE. Bacterial contamination of drip sets. *N Z Med J* 1973; 77: 390–391.

22. Woodside W, Woodside WM, D'Arcy EM, *et al.* Intravenous infusions as vehicles for infection. *Pharm J* 1975; 215: 606.

23. Deeks EN, Natsios FA. Contamination of infusion fluids by bacteria and fungi during preparation and administration. *Am J Hosp Pharm* 1971; 28: 764–767.

24. D'Arcy PF, Woodside ME. Drug additives, a potential source of bacterial contamination of infusion fluids. *Lancet* 1973; ii: 96.

25. Queria RA, Hiels SW, Klimek JJ, *et al.* Bacteriologic contamination of intravenous infusion delivery systems in an intensive care unit. *Am J Med* 1986; 80: 364–368.

26. Jahnte M. Use of the HACCP concept for the risk analysis of pharmaceutical manufacturing processes. *Eur J Parent Sci* 1997; 2(4): 113–117.

27. NHS Executive. *Clinical Governance: Quality in the New NHS (HSC 99/065)*. London: Department of Health, 1999.

28. Lee MG, Oldcorne MA, personal communication.

29. Anonymous. *Note for Guidance on the Maximum Shelf Life for Sterile Products for Human Use after First Opening*. London: Committee for Proprietary Medicinal Products; European Medicines Evaluation Agency, 1998.

30. Brown S, Baker MH. The sterility testing of dispensed radiopharmaceuticals. *Nucl Med Commun* 1986; 7: 327–366.

31. Abra RM, Bell NDS, Horton PW. The growth of micro-organisms in some parenteral radiopharmaceuticals. *Int J Pharmaceutics* 1980; 5: 187–193.

32. Francomb MM, Ford JL, Hunt P, *et al.* Investigations of antimicrobial action of cytotoxic drugs at concentrations used in bolus therapy. *Pharm J* 1990; R38.

33. Weil DC, Arnow PM. Safety of refrigerated storage of admixed parenteral fluids. *J Clin Microbiol* 1988; 26: 1787–1790.

34. Mehta DK. *British National Formulary.* Current edition. London: British Medical Association and Royal Pharmaceutical Society of Great Britain.

35. Royal Pharmaceutical Society. *Medicines, Ethics and Practice: A Guide for Pharmacists.* Current edition. London: Royal Pharmaceutical Society of Great Britain.

36. *Environmental Cleanliness in Enclosed Spaces. BS 5295:1989.* Milton Keynes: British Standards Institute, 1989.

37. *Clean Rooms and Associated Controlled Environments Part 1: Classification of Air Cleanliness. BS EN ISO 14644-1:1999.* London: British Standards Institute, 1999.

38. Lee MG, Midcalf B, eds. *Isolators for Pharmaceutical Applications*. Cambridge: HMSO, 1995.

39. *The Ionising Radiation (Medical Exposure) Regulations. SI 2000 No.1059; 2000.*

40. Parenteral Society. *Environmental Contamination Control Practice: Technical Monograph No. 2*. Swindon: Parenteral Society, 1989.

41. Parenteral Drug Association. *Validation of Aseptic Filling for Solution Drug Products: Technical Monograph No. 2*. Maryland: Parenteral Drug Association, 1980.

42. Needle R, Sizer T, eds. *The CIVAS Handbook*. London: Pharmaceutical Press, 1998.

43. *Microbiological Safety Cabinets. BS 5726:1992*. Milton Keynes: British Standards Institute, 1992.

44. *The Quality Assurance of Radiopharmaceuticals*, 3rd edn. Joint Working Party of UK Radiopharmacy Group and the NHS Pharmaceutical Quality Control Committee, 2000.

45. Murthough SM, Hiom SJ, Palmer M, *et al*. A survey of disinfectant use in hospital pharmacy aseptic preparation areas. *Pharm J* 2000; 264: 446–448.

46. British Pharmacopoeia Commission Secretariat. *British Pharmacopoeia*. Current edition. London: HMSO.

47. Institute of Sterile Services Management. *CSSD – Quality Standards and Recommended Practices for Sterile Services Departments*. Truro: Institute of Sterile Services Management, 1998.

48. *Clean Steam for Sterilisation. HTM 2031*. Leeds: NHS Estates, 1997.

49. *Control of Substances Hazardous to Health Regulations. SI 1657; 1988.*

50. *Transport of Dangerous Goods (Safety Advisers) Regulations. SI 257; 1999.*

51. *Carriage of Dangerous Goods by Road Regulations. SI 2095; 1996.*

52. *The Radioactive Material (Road Transport) (Great Britain) Regulations. SI 1350; 1996.*

53. *Quality Audits and Their Application to Hospital Pharmacy Technical Services*. NHS Pharmaceutical Quality Control Committee, 1999.

54. Validation. In: Lund W, ed. *The Pharmaceutical Codex*, 12th edn. London: Pharmaceutical Press, 1994: 389–398.

55. Parenteral Society. *The Use of Process Simulation Tests in the Evaluation of Processes for the Manufacture of Sterile Products: Technical Monograph No. 4*. Swindon: Parenteral Society, 1993.

56. *Detection Methods for Chemical Contaminants*. London: NHS Pharmaceutical Quality Control Committee, 1996.

57. *The TickIT Guide, Issue 4. ISO 9002*. London: British Standards Institute, 1998.

58. Institute of Electrical and Electronics Engineers. *IEEE Standard for Software Verification and Validation; IEEE Std 1012-1998*. Piscataway, NJ: Institute of Electrical and Electronics Engineers, 1998.

59. Institute of Electrical and Electronics Engineers. *Supplement to IEEE Standard for Software Verification and Validation: Content Map to IEEE/EIA 12207.1-1997; IEEE Std 1012A-1998*. Piscataway, NJ: Institute of Electrical and Electronics Engineers, 1998.

60. *Good Automated Manufacturing Practice (GAMP 3): GAMP Guide for Validation of Automated Systems in Pharmaceutical Manufacture; Vol 1, Part 1: User Guide; Vol 1, Part 2: Supplier Guide; Vol 2: Best Practice for Users and Suppliers*. Belgium: ISPE European Office, 1999.

Useful addresses

Publications of The Parenteral Society, the British Standards Institute and the NHS Quality Control Committee are available from the addresses below:

The Parenteral Society
99 Ermin Street
Stratton St Margaret
Swindon
Wilts SN3 4NL

British Standards Institute
389 Chiswick High Road
London W4 4AL

Secretary to NHS Pharmaceutical Quality Control Committee
Mr M Knowles
Pharmacy Department
Guy's Hospital
St Thomas Street
London SE1 9RT

Index

Page numbers in **bold** refer to the main discussion of a topic; page numbers in *italics* refer to tables.